CARDIAC DRUG SAFETY
A Bench to Bedside Approach

CARDIAC
DRUG
SAFETY

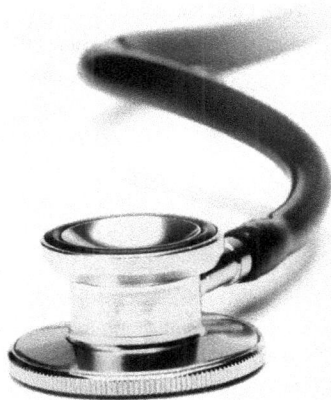

A Bench to Bedside Approach

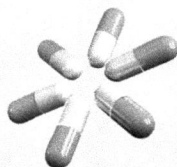

Matthew J Killeen
University of Cambridge, UK

World Scientific

NEW JERSEY · LONDON · SINGAPORE · BEIJING · SHANGHAI · HONG KONG · TAIPEI · CHENNAI

Published by

World Scientific Publishing Co. Pte. Ltd.

5 Toh Tuck Link, Singapore 596224

USA office: 27 Warren Street, Suite 401-402, Hackensack, NJ 07601

UK office: 57 Shelton Street, Covent Garden, London WC2H 9HE

British Library Cataloguing-in-Publication Data
A catalogue record for this book is available from the British Library.

CARDIAC DRUG SAFETY
A Bench to Bedside Approach

ISBN-13 978-981-4317-45-0
ISBN-10 981-4317-45-4

Typeset by Stallion Press
Email: enquiries@stallionpress.com

Printed in Singapore.

Contents

Foreword

"Et causae quoque aestimatio saepe morbum solvit"*
[Celsus: Prooemium 69, De Medicina]

The academic legitimacy and relevance of a biomedical discipline ultimately depends upon its eventual applicability to improving human health. Such a vindication is emerging for the exciting recent developments in the cell physiology of ion channel function, and the spread of their resulting electric currents both within and between cells both in isolated organs and intact organisms. The resulting analytical and quantitative, rather than merely descriptive, understanding of electrophysiological processes within the working heart has proven clearly translatable to understanding and management in the clinically important area of cardiac arrhythmias, a major public health burden.

This book, directed at electrophysiological applications in the particular area of cardiac drug safety specifically in relationship to potential serious cardiac arrhythmic effects of therapeutic agents, is particularly timely. This area has become critical to discovery pipelines

---

* A consideration of the cause often explains the disease.

for pharmacotherapeutic agents in relationship to the safety of their clinical use, whether by themselves or in combination with other clinical manoeuvres or particular pre-existing clinical conditions. This important and topical area is critically covered with scientific rigour and practically useful scholarship. The author uniquely combines a successful electrophysiological benchside background within the cardiac arrhythmia field with his current activities in the areas of pharmaceutical development and its financial and regulatory implications. His approach firmly begins from clearly formulated scientific fundamentals based on recent developments in our understanding of ion channel function and the resulting myocyte excitation and its propagation. This underpins coverage of the clinical and physiological features of cardiac arrhythmias and their initiation by pharmacological agents. These in turn lead to critical assessments of preclinical methods for assessing potential arrhythmic effects. The treatment then extends into important new areas in pediatric drug safety and atrial fibrillation, before gathering the field of ideas into a discussion of possible ways forward towards ensuring cardiac drug electrophysiological safety.

This book thus bridges the benchside and the clinical science and their implications for drug discovery and evaluation. Through tight but lucid exposition and well-placed examples, it clarifies each of the areas involved and their interrelationships within this strategic interdisciplinary field. It does so in a manner accessible to audiences whether working within the scientific, industrial or financial aspects of drug discovery and development. It deserves the widest possible readership and every success.

Christopher Huang DM (Oxford), ScD (Cambridge), FSB
Professor of Cell Physiology
Physiological Laboratory, and Department of Biochemistry
and Professorial Fellow of Murray Edwards College
University of Cambridge
Independent Nonexecutive Director and Chairman
Technical Committee
Hutchison China Meditech
Director, Cambridge Cardiac Systems

Preface

In the past decade, cardiovascular safety has emerged as a critical factor shaping the development, approval, and commercial potential of a wide array of novel pharmaceutical products. Prompted by several cases of recalls due to potentially lethal cardiac arrhythmias, regulatory bodies now require developers to conduct a battery of safety tests during a drug's journey to the market. The introduction of these safety measures represent an important milestone in the pharmaceutical industry's history and have helped to ensure increased patient safety.

Although there are many detailed books on cardiac safety and drug-induced arrhythmias, most have been written for a specialist audience. However, the increased emphasis on a new medical product's cardiac safety exposes an increasing number of individuals, in many different functions, to this pivotal drug safety phenomenon. One of the overarching aims of this book is, therefore, to demystify drug-induced arrhythmias by explaining how these events may arise, how the cardiac safety of new medical products is tested, and what drug safety challenges remain for the pharmaceutical industry. Using a first principles approach to understanding this adverse event, this book begins with an introduction to cardiac electrophysiology, arrhythmia mechanisms, and clinical arrhythmia syndromes. These preliminary sections introduce several fundamental concepts of cardiac physiology that are essential for understanding drug-induced proarrhythmia. Later sections examine several case studies of drugs that were shown to evoke arrhythmias in patients and how the safety profiles of new drugs are evaluated during preclinical and clinical development.

The field of cardiac safety is continuously evolving; new drug safety biomarkers, potentially disruptive technologies, novel concepts of safety testing, and increasing knowledge of other cardiac adverse events are challenging the current drug safety paradigm. As such, another core aim of this book is to examine what the future might hold for the field of cardiac safety and to identify several areas of remaining unmet need. Later chapters of the book explore drug-induced arrhythmias in pediatric patients and drug-induced atrial fibrillation. In taking an exploratory approach to discussing these emerging areas in cardiac safety, it is my intention to provide readers with an understanding of the challenges remaining in this field and what some of the future areas of focus might be.

Many people have greatly influenced my interest in, and understanding of, cardiac safety, and I am indebted to them for their inspiration and support. Christopher Huang first introduced me to the exciting, yet challenging, field of cardiac electrophysiology; he has been a constant source of encouragement and he continues to drive my passion for this area. I am also extremely grateful to Andrew Grace, Calum Macrae, and Glyn Thomas who, with their vast experience in clinical cardiology, played a central role in my understanding of clinical arrhythmia syndromes. I have also been fortunate enough to work alongside several cardiac safety experts through the Cardiac Safety Research Consortium. In particular I wish to thank John Finkle, Mitchell Krucoff, Gary Gintant, Boaz Mendzelevski, and Philip Sager for their invaluable insight and support. I am also grateful to Joy Quek, at World Scientific Press, for her help throughout this project. Finally I am indebted to my wife, Katherine Linder, who has played a pivotal role in this project. Through her tireless encouragement, enthusiasm, and support Katherine has made writing this book a considerable pleasure.

Dr. Matthew J. Killeen
London, 2011

CHAPTER 1

Challenges Facing the Pharmaceutical Industry in the 21st Century

Introduction

In the past decade, the classical drug discovery model has been, and continues to be, challenged. Within the past 12 years, the pharmaceutical industry as a whole has experienced a worrying trend; the number of new chemical entities (NCEs) approved by regulatory agencies has gradually decreased. The number of NCE approvals by the United States Food and Drug Administration (FDA) has declined from 35 in 1997 to 16 in 2010 (Figure 1); between January 1997 and December 2009, new drug approvals hit lows of around 15 per year in 2002 and 2005–2007.

In order to move potentially life-saving new products through the regulatory process in a shorter period of time, the FDA has developed certain methods of expediting regulatory approval for NCEs that address serious unmet medical needs: Accelerated Approval, Fast Track product development, and Priority Review. Accelerated Approval allows companies to either use a surrogate end point of efficacy in clinical trials, or to limit the potential safety concerns of new medications by restricting their use to controlled patient populations; compounds entering Fast Track product development must be targeted towards life-threatening illnesses, thereby satisfying important unmet medical needs. NCEs

1

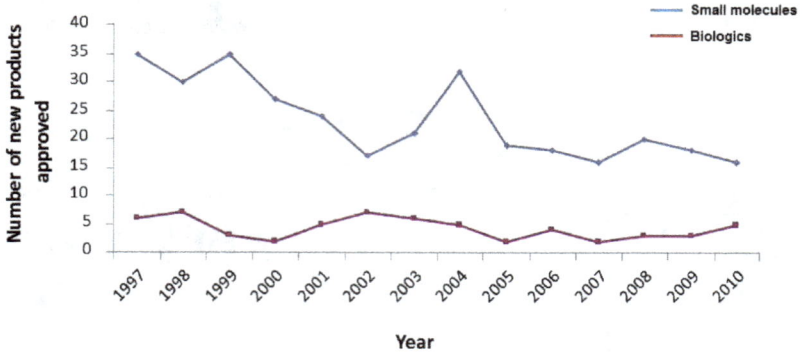

Figure 1:   Small molecule and biologic drug approvals by the FDA between 1997 and 2010.

Sources: FDA and independent analysis.

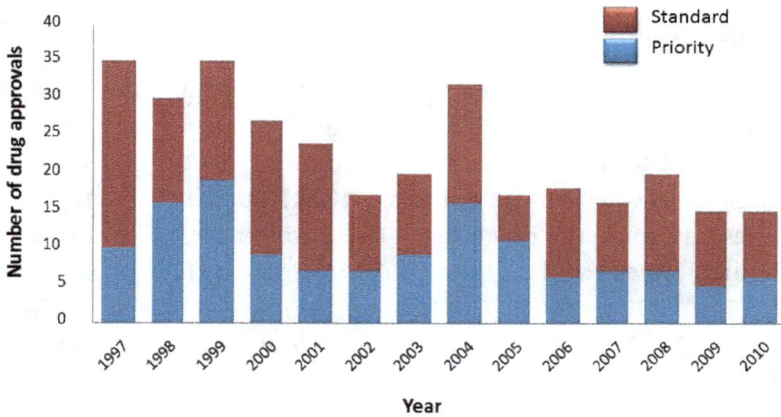

Figure 2:   Priority and standard drug approvals by the FDA between 1997 and 2010.

Sources: FDA and independent analysis.

undergoing Priority Reviews can expect shorter decision times from the FDA upon submission of a completed application. Figure 2 shows the number of NCE standard and priority drug review approvals by the FDA between 1997–2009. Compared with the data from 1997, the number of approvals by both the standard and priority review processes significantly decreased in 2010, particularly so for standard approvals, which fell by 64% (Figure 3).

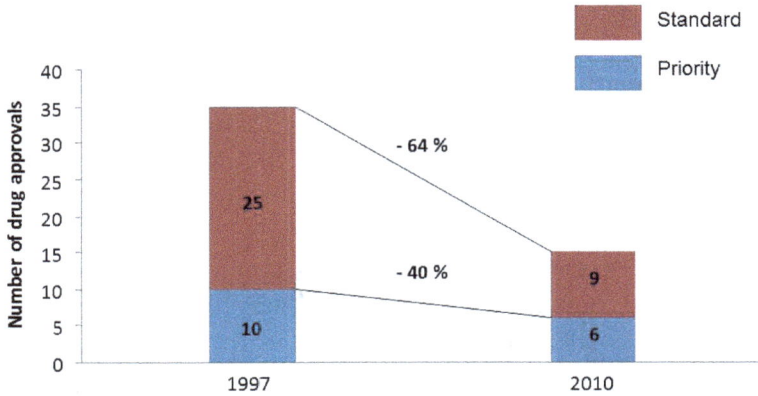

Figure 3: A comparison between the number of FDA priority and standard drug approvals in 1997 and 2010.

Sources: FDA and independent analysis.

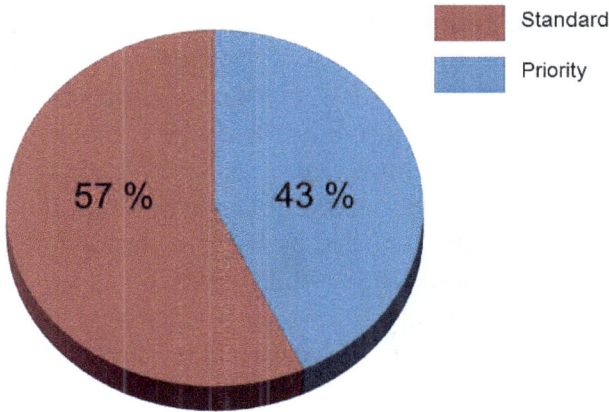

Figure 4: The proportion of FDA priority and standard drug approvals between 1997 and 2010.

Sources: FDA and independent analysis.

However, when taking the average number of approvals by these two, distinct regulatory mechanisms, standard approvals still account for the majority of total FDA drug approvals (57% versus 43%; Figure 4).

An explanation that is often put forward to account for the reduced number of drug approvals is "declining research and development productivity" in major biopharmaceutical companies. However, such explanations are hard to reconcile with our significantly increased knowledge of human physiology, pharmacology and disease mechanisms over the past 50 years. Furthermore, these advances have been coupled with ever more sophisticated drug discovery and development techniques, and accompanying manufacturing processes.

The pharmaceutical industry is responding to this environment by a number of different mechanisms. Firstly, companies are broadening their therapeutic strategies by entering into new disease sectors, such as cancer and neurodegenerative diseases, which have traditionally been the territory of the biotechnology industry. Secondly, companies are reducing their level of activity in crowded therapeutic sectors that often demand significantly reduced pricing of new products and a strong, and ultimately expensive, marketing strategy to generate demand amongst health care providers. Although entry into the biotechnology sector provides the pharmaceutical industry with a number of distinct advantages, such as a reduced threat of generic competition and an ability to command higher prices for approved treatments, it is important for the industry to bear in mind that as a whole, biotechnology companies have generated lower profits compared to traditional pharmaceutical companies. A powerful analysis of profitability of the biotechnology industry conducted by Harvard Business School reveals that between 1975 and 2004 while revenue soared, profitability remained negligible (Pisano, 2006). In fact, in 2004 the majority of publicly held biotechnology companies had negative cash flows, and of the companies that did have positive cash flows, 15 companies accounted for the majority of the income generated.

The Impact of Cardiac Toxicity on the Pharmaceutical Industry

The safety of new medications acting through both familiar and novel mechanisms of action remains a critical concern for the pharmaceutical industry. As such, stringent preclinical and clinical safety studies are warranted prior to drug approval by regulatory agencies. Following approval, post-marketing surveillance initiatives track drug-induced adverse even:s; events can be reported by prescribing physicians or directly to regulatory agencies. In the United States, for example, MedWatch is the FDA's drug safety reporting program, and it provides both physicians and patients with up-to-date drug safety and product recall information on medications currently marketed in the United States. The number of pharmaceutical product safety alerts issued by the FDA has been steadily increasing since 2002; 85 pharmaceutical safety alerts were reported in 2009 and documented by MedWatch, compared to 36 in 2002, representing a 136% increase (Figure 5). Such a trend could result from a number of different factors including: (1) improved awareness of the range of adverse events that can be induced by medications; (2) improved understanding of the definition of a drug-induced adverse event; (3) improved physician and patient awareness of adverse events; and (4) more sophisticated and efficient reporting procedures. Nevertheless these safety alert data indicate that drug safety in the major pharmaceutical markets is becoming an increasingly important issue.

From January 1990 through August 2009, 41 pharmaceutical products were withdrawn from the major pharmaceutical markets

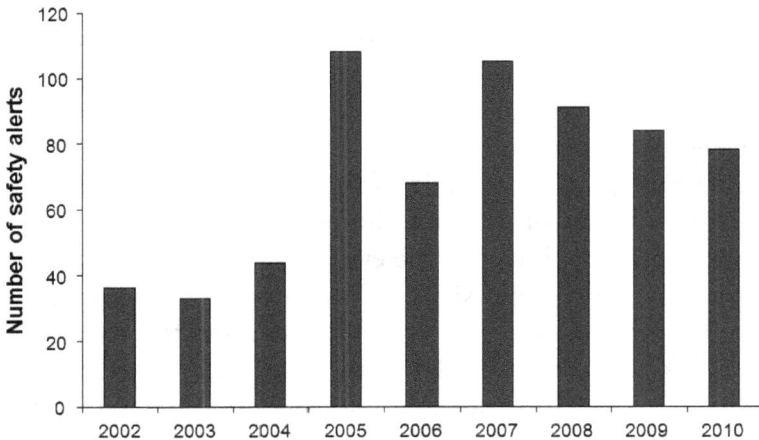

Figure 5: Number of drug safety alerts received by the FDA between 2002 and 2010.
Sources: FDA MedWatch and independent analysis.

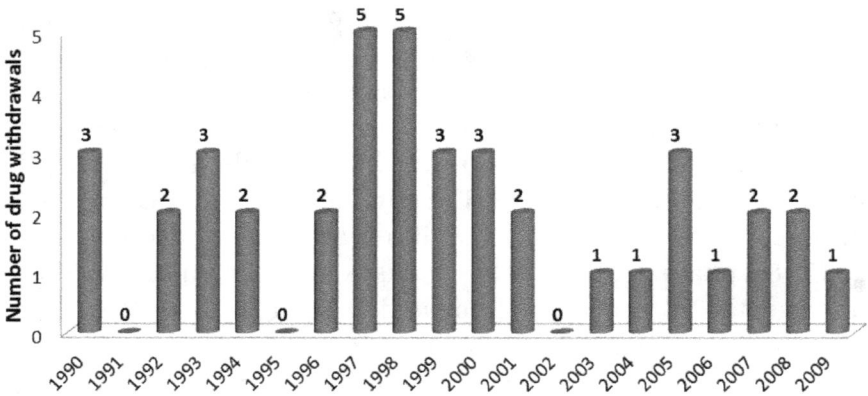

Figure 6: Number of pharmaceutical products withdrawn from major pharmaceutical markets, due to safety concerns, between 1990 and 2009.

Sources: FDA and independent analysis.

following reports of serious adverse events (Figure 6). Product recalls in the latter half of the decade were lower (16 from 2000–2009, compared to 22 between 1990 and 2000), which could reflect improved drug safety screening programs that have become commonplace following high-profile major product recalls occurring between 1998 and 2004. Collectively, drug safety alerts, product recalls, and improved knowledge of potential adverse events can have multiple significant consequences upon the pharmaceutical and health care communities alike. In the case of a currently marketed medication, fear of drug-induced unwanted effects could lead to reduced patient compliance with a medication or reduced physician prescribing of potentially life-saving medications. For the pharmaceutical industry, the withdrawal of a major product may foster a negative public image in the eyes of the patient and health care professional, which could significantly impact sales of drugs acting via similar mechanisms of action. Furthermore, the recall of rofecoxib (Vioxx), a non-steroidal anti-inflammatory agent (NSAID) towards the end of 2004, for example, was associated with a significant fall in the share closing price of the drug's developer, from U.S. $45.09 on 2 September 2004 to U.S. $26.8 on 2 November 2004 (Figure 7).

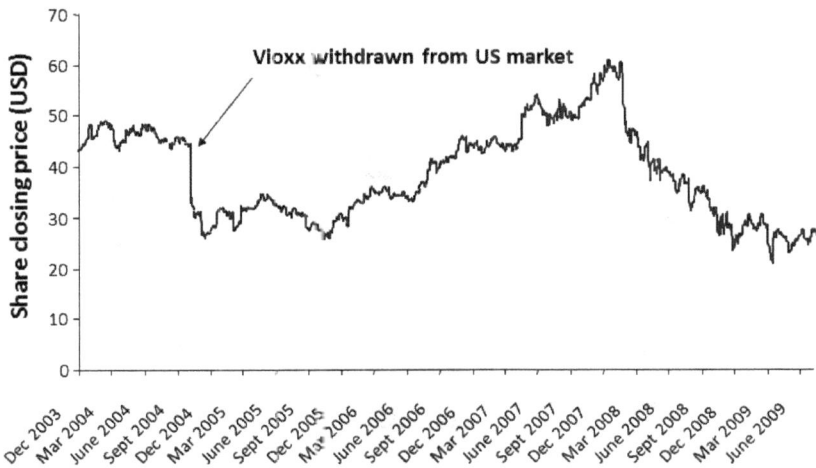

Figure 7:   The effect of a drug recall, due to a major adverse cardiac event, on a company's share price.

Pharmaceutical products that have been withdrawn following reports of serious adverse events have been targeted towards a range of therapeutic areas; the two associated with the highest number of recalls, however, are products acting on the neurological and cardiovascular systems, which account for 39% and 14% of all recalls, respectively (Figure 8). However, such trends may not necessarily reflect inherent toxicological profiles of pharmaceutical products targeting these two therapy areas. Increasing knowledge and awareness of neurological disorders, such as depression and schizophrenia, for example, could have catalyzed increased drug discovery efforts in this therapeutic sector, thereby increasing the likelihood of adverse events to be associated with neurological medications. In the case of cardiovascular drugs, a number of factors could drive their high rate of adverse events such as the presence of existing cardiovascular conditions in patients (an important risk factor for drug-induced toxicity) and in many cases their intentional effects on the heart which, as discussed below, is one of the organ systems most commonly affected by drug toxicity.

Analysis of the types of adverse events reported with withdrawn medications reveals that three major physiological systems are

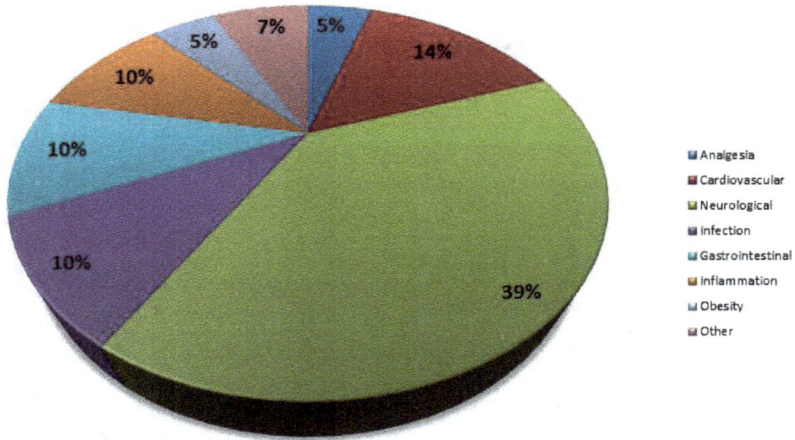

Figure 8: The therapeutic indications of drugs withdrawn from major pharmaceutical markets due to safety concerns.

predominantly affected: the renal, hepatic, and cardiovascular systems (Figure 9). Cardiovascular adverse events account for the majority of safety concerns associated with pharmaceutical products withdrawn between January 1990 and August 2009. Drug-induced QT prolongation (reflecting profound disturbances in the heart's electrical properties) and the risk of potentially lethal cardiac arrhythmias has been associated with 50% of all products withdrawn from the major markets due to cardiovascular safety concerns (Figure 10).

Market withdrawals of pharmaceutical products following reports of drug-induced QT prolongation and cardiac arrhythmias have had significant financial implications for pharmaceutical companies. For example, Table 1 lists six drugs withdrawn since 1997 due to concerns over their ability to induce cardiac arrhythmias in patients.

If terfenadine, astemizole, cisapride, sertindole, and geprafloxacin continued to generate similar sales for a further 12 months as they did in the year before their withdrawal, it can be estimated that the recall of these products has cost the industry at least U.S. $1.7 billion in lost sales. These amounts are based on the assumption that the

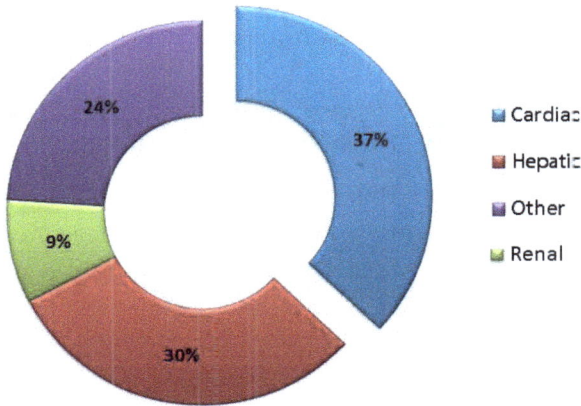

Figure 9: Major adverse events that have evoked drug withdrawals.

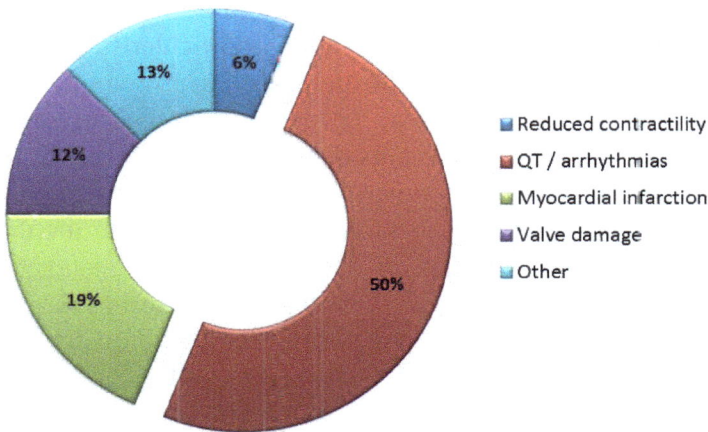

Figure 10: Cardiac adverse events that have evoked drug withdrawals.

listed drugs continued to generate the same level of revenue, which is dependent upon a range of factors such as the level of competition in the marketplace and the position of the product within its respective life cycle. Cisapride, for example, was removed from the market just six years after its launch and potentially before it had achieved maximal market penetration and its peak sales potential. Including mibefradil, which analysts had predicted would garner sales of up to

Table 1:   Select Drugs Removed from Major Pharmaceutical Markets Due to Their Risk QT Prolongation and Proarrhythmia and Their Sales in the Year Prior to Their Withdrawal.

Drug Name	Year Withdrawn	Final Year Sales Prior to Withdrawal ($ Millions)
Terfenadine	1998	600
Mibefradil	1998	2900 (projected sales estimate)
Sertindole	1998	15.6
Astemizole	1999	90
Geprafloxacin	1999	23.5
Cispride	2000	950

U.S. $2.9 billion, the total loss to the pharmaceutical industry from just these six drugs could exceed U.S. $4.5 billion.

Drug-induced cardiac adverse events, particularly QT prolongation and proarrhythmia, can therefore have major economic implications for pharmaceutical companies. However, predicting the risk of these major adverse events occurring in large patient populations, following a drug's approval, poses several major challenges to developers. The purpose of this book is to closely examine the clinical features of drug-induced arrhythmias, explore the mechanisms underlying such potentially devastating events, and assess some of the current methods used by the pharmaceutical industry to profile the cardiac safety of new therapies. Additionally, several emerging cardiac safety concepts, and their potential implications to drug development are also described.

References

Pisano, G. (2006). *Science Business: The Promise, the Reality, and the Future of Biotech.* Harvard Business School Press, Boston.

CHAPTER 2

The Cellular Basis of Cardiac Electrophysiology

Introduction

Each contraction of the heart pumps blood throughout the body to sustain vital physiological functions. The heart is an electrically-excitable organ and each heart beat is initiated and controlled by intrinsic electrical impulses that trigger the heart's rhythmic contractions. These highly coordinated electrical impulses, known as action potentials (APs), are controlled by cardiac ion channels. Abnormalities in ion channel function lead to electrical instability and are a fundamental cause of cardiac arrhythmias, including those induced by drugs. By closely examining the ion channels underlying the cardiac AP, and its relationship to the electrocardiogram (ECG), this chapter discusses some of the most important components of cardiac electrophysiology that will serve as a basis for understanding many of the cardiac drug safety concepts introduced in later chapters, including how arrhythmias arise and how they can be detected.

The Initiation of the Heart Beat

The initiation of each heart beat begins with an electrical impulse that is discharged from a small area of tissue in the right atrium, the sino atrial node, which comprises specialized pacemaker cells. This

11

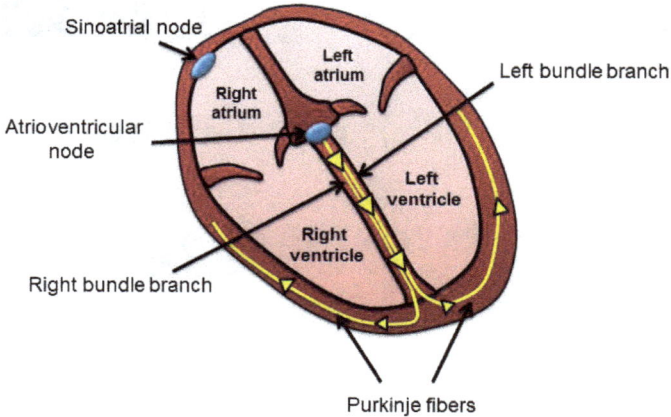

Figure 1: **The cardiac conduction system.**

impulse then propagates through the left and right atria, causing contraction of these chambers of the heart and forcing blood into the left and right ventricles, respectively. The electrical impulse then arrives to the atrioventricular node and, after a brief pause, it is rapidly conducted through the left and right bundle branches to the Purkinje fibers, at which point it activates the left and right ventricles, causing them to contract and to pump blood to different regions of the body (the conduction of electrical impulses that mediate the contraction of the heart is illustrated in Figure 1). Disruptions to this tightly regulated process, which may arise due to disease or the adverse effects of drugs, can lead to the development of electrical instability within the heart which may in turn give rise to potentially lethal uncoordinated contractions of the heart mediated by aberrant electrical activity (cardiac arrhythmias).

The Ventricular Cardiac Action Potential

The ventricular AP represents the combined coordinated electrical activity of a wide range of cardiac ion channels existing in open or closed states. The duration of the action potential represents the time taken for the heart to return to a resting state (a process termed repolarization) following its initial activation (depolarization) which pumps blood throughout the body. In the human ventricular cardiac AP, the rapid upstroke phase (Phase 0) marks depolarization which is caused by the opening of voltage-sensitive Na^+ channels resulting in a large influx of Na^+ ions into cardiac cells (myocytes); these positively charged ions entering a cardiac myocyte raise its membrane potential and initiate a series of other electrical and physiological processes in the heart. After briefly opening, Na^+ channels rapidly close and a small outward repolarizing K^+ current results in a brief period of repolarization due to the efflux of positively charged K^+ ions from the myocyte; this transient period of partial repolarization is known as Phase 1 on the cardiac AP. Calcium channels (the L-type Ca^{2+} channel) subsequently open and give rise to Ca^{2+} influx (Phase 2 on the cardiac action potential) which in turn causes further Ca^{2+} release from the myocyte's intracellular Ca^{2+} store (the sarcoplasmic reticulum), in a process referred to as calcium-induced-calcium release (CICR) which initiates the coordinated contraction of the heart. As the L-type Ca^{2+} channels close, a large outward K^+ current conducted through major repolarizing K^+ channels gives rise to the AP's repolarization phase (Phase 3) in which the myocyte's membrane potential returns to its resting state in preparation for the next depolarization of the heart (Phase 4 on the cardiac AP). These ion channels and their roles in cardiac excitation and the AP are illustrated in Figure 2.

The expression levels of cardiac ion channels vary considerably in different regions of the heart, particularly in the ventricle; this gives rise to ventricular APs of varying morphologies and durations that are considered to play an important role in establishing a regular, coordinated cardiac rhythm. The waveform of the ventricular AP is also species-dependent, owing in part to physiological differences in heart rate and different expression patterns of cardiac ion channels. The morphologies of human and mouse ventricular APs, for example, are compared in Figure 3.

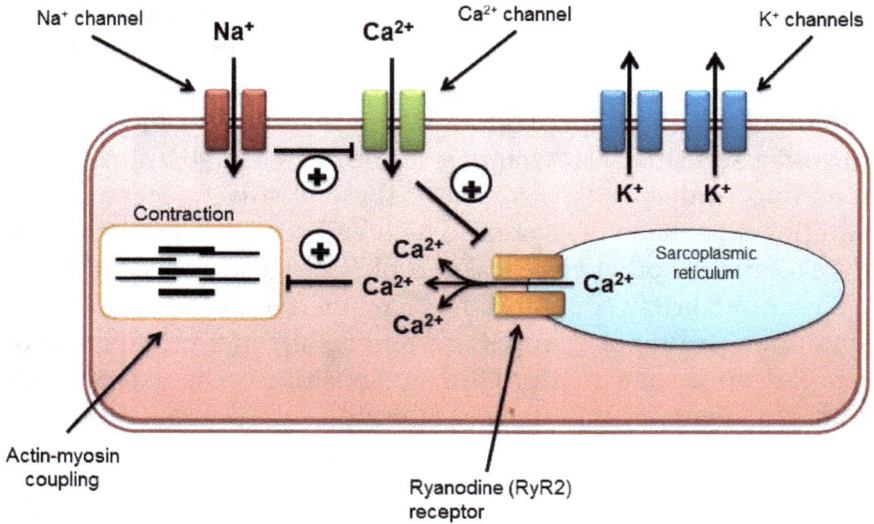

Figure 2:   Key components of a cardiac myocyte that regulate depolarization, muscle contraction, and repolarization.

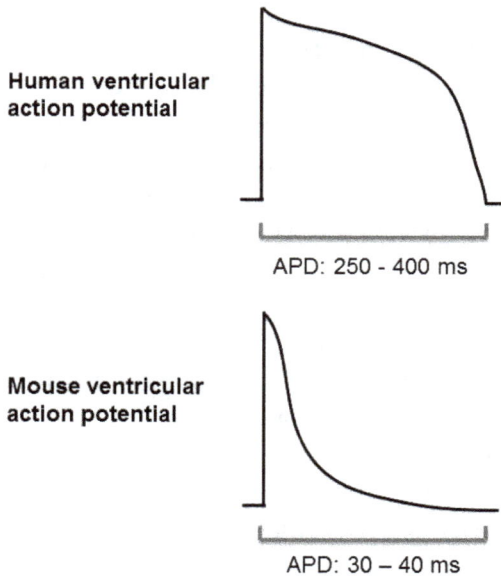

Figure 3:   A comparison between human and mouse ventricular action potential morphologies. APD = Action potential duration.

The Relationship Between the Cardiac Action Potential and the Electrocardiogram

The electrocardiogram (ECG) is a measure of the heart's electrical activity that is recorded from the body's surface via a series of electrodes. The electrical activity underlying each heart beat is captured by the ECG; the small P wave represents depolarization of the atria, the much larger QRS complex represents depolarization of the ventricles, and the T wave reflects repolarization of the ventricles — the end of the T wave marks the point at which the ventricles are completely repolarized and in a resting state in anticipation of the next depolarizing electrical impulse from the sinoatrial node. In this regard, the time between the Q wave of the QRS complex and the end of the T wave, a measurement known as the QT interval, reflects the time taken for the ventricles to repolarize following their depolarization and is therefore a marker of the ventricular cardiac AP duration (APD) (Figure 4). The ECG is a fundamental diagnostic tool for the physician and distinct changes in the ECG waveform can indicate a wide range of pathologies, particularly delays in repolarization, indicated by prolongation of the QT interval, induced by drugs or disease.

The following sections describe in further detail the core cardiac ion channels and the depolarizing and repolarizing ionic currents that they mediate to govern the rhythmic contractions of the heart.

Ion Channels Underlying the Cardiac Action Potential

Sodium channels

Voltage-sensitive Na^+ channels are an essential component to the cardiac AP, opening rapidly following membrane depolarization, and comprising Phase 0 of the AP, and closing just as quickly to ensure a prompt termination of the electrical signal. The rapid influx of Na^+ ions into cardiac myocytes initiates a chain of events which ultimately lead to the coordinated contraction and relaxation of cardiac muscle and the propagation of electrical signals throughout the heart. Each Na^+ channel is comprised of a pore forming alpha-subunit and possibly one or two auxillary beta-subunits. The alpha-subunit of cardiac

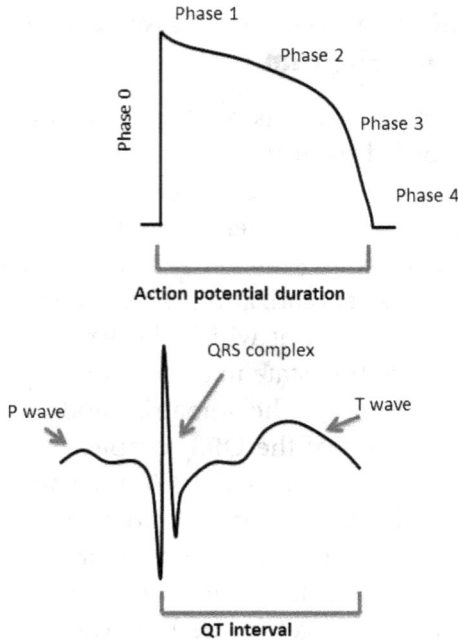

Figure 4: A comparison between the human ventricular action potential and the ECG illustrating how the APD can be viewed as a marker of the QT interval.

Na$^+$ channels is known as Nav1.5 and is encoded by the SCN5a gene. The alpha-subunit consists of four repeats (domains I–IV) of a six membrane-spanning protein. Membrane spanning segments of each domain are labeled S1–S6, where S4 comprises the channel's voltage sensor and S5–S6 regions form the pore of the Na$^+$ channel through which Na$^+$ ions enter cardiac myocytes. A functional Na$^+$ channel therefore contains four voltage sensors and four pore-forming segments. The S4 voltage sensor present in each domain responds to changes in voltage by physically moving upwards in an anticlockwise direction. This movement results in a conformational change in the Na$^+$ channel, which opens the channel's pore (channel activation) and allows Na$^+$ ions to enter the myocyte.

Activation of Na$^+$ channels is immediately followed by inactivation. This is mediated by a cytoplasmic linker between domains III and IV that consists of three amino acid residues (isoleucine, phenylalanine and methionine; known as the IFM motif). Within a matter of milliseconds, the IFM motif can plug the inner pore region of the Na^+ channel and lead to inactivation and closing of the channel. Inactivation of the channel is dependent upon repolarization of the myocyte; repolarization to the resting membrane potential removes the IFM motif from the inner pore of the channel, which in turn transitions to the closed state where it is once again able to reopen in the event of membrane depolarization.

During the ensuing plateau phase of the AP, it is estimated that 99% of Na^+ channels are in a closed state, whereas approximately 1% of channels remain open and mediate a small persistent inward current that plays an important role in counteracting strong repolarizing K^+ currents. Studies of long QT syndrome (a genetic cardiac disease that can lead to arrhythmias) type 3 have highlighted the pathological consequences of a large number of Na^+ channels remaining in the activated state throughout the AP due to abnormal Na^+ channel inactivation. In this disease a mutation disrupts Na^+ channel inactivation and leads to a persistent Na^+ current in which channels fail to inactivate. Such effects can lead to the generation of lethal ventricular arrhythmias.

Accessory subunits for Na^+ channels have been identified which modulate the channel's expression, inactivation properties and current density; these are known as SCN1b, SCN2b, and SCN3b. Recently, the SCN3b subunit has been linked to a range of cardiac electrical abnormalities. Mice genetically engineered to lack SCN3b, have slower heart rates, longer PR intervals and shortened ventricular APDs. The absence of SCN3b also results in a significant reduction in Na^+ current and a high susceptibility to atrial and ventricular arrhythmias.

Calcium channels

Voltage-sensitive Ca^{2+} channels are classified according to their thresholds for activation: high-voltage-activated (HVA) and low-voltage-activated (LVA). Only HVA channels are present in cardiac myocytes. HVA channels can be further subdivided: L- (long lasting), N- (neither), P- (Purkinje), Q- and R- (remaining), with the L-type Ca^{2+} channel (LTCC) constituting voltage-dependent Ca^{2+} influx through HVA Ca^{2+} channels in ventricular myocytes. LTCCs are activated by depolarization and they generate an inward Ca^{2+} current which in turn causes a large release of Ca^{2+} from internal stores via the ryanodine (RyR) receptor. This process is termed CICR (Fabiato and Fabiato, 1972) and it initiates myocardial contraction, pumping blood throughout the body. Increases in intracellular Ca^{2+} levels can also activate a broad range of enzymes. Of these, the role of calcium calmodulin (CaM) kinase type II has been studied in relation to its possible role in cardiac arrhythmias (Anderson, 2004; Wu *et al.*, 2002). Increases in intracellular Ca^{2+} activate CaM kinase type II (CaMKII) which can increase the open probability of LTCCs which may in turn give rise to arrhythmogenic inward currents.

Calcium channels do not open immediately in response to membrane depolarization; their opening is delayed relative to Na^+ channels and, as such, they do not largely contribute to phase 0 of the cardiac AP. In addition to mediating contraction, influx of Ca^{2+} through Ca^{2+} channels opposes outward K^+ currents and forms the plateau phase of the AP. Nevertheless, Ca^{2+} channels do inactivate rapidly through Ca^{2+}-dependent channel inactivation mechanisms, which terminate the AP plateau phase and permit complete repolarization to take place.

Voltage-sensitive Ca^{2+} channels are structurally similar to voltage-sensitive Na^+ channels: the alpha-subunit is comprised of four domains (I–IV), with each domain possessing an S4 voltage sensor and S5 and S6 pore forming regions. The Ca^{2+} channel alpha-subunit protein is known as Cav1.2a and it is encoded by the CACNA1C gene. Auxiliary subunits have been identified for voltage-sensitive Ca^{2+} channels. Intracellular beta-subunits increase current density when co-expressed with alpha-subunits either through increasing the open probability of the channels or by increasing the density of alpha-subunits in the plasma membrane (Yamaguchi *et al.*, 1998). Additionally, transmembrane $\alpha_2\delta$ subunits modulate Ca^{2+} channel activation, inactivation and current amplitudes (Bangalore *et al.*, 1996).

Potassium channels

Potassium (K^+) channels are present in virtually all cell types of all organisms where they serve a multitude of biological functions by exerting a dampening effect on cell functions. In contrast to Na^+ and Ca^{2+} channels, there exists a great deal more diversity of K^+ channels. Open K^+ channels diminish cellular excitability. The first voltage-sensitive K^+ channel cloned was the *Shaker* K^+ channel from the fruit fly *Drosophila*, so called because under ether anesthesia the fly would shake its legs. Additional K^+ channels were later cloned from the *Drosophila* and were termed *Shal*, *Shaw* and *Shab*, each representing a single gene. However, there are significantly more channels encoded by the mammalian equivalent of *Drosophila Shaker*, *Shal*, *Shaw* and *Shab* genes, representing a great deal of evolutionary diversification. In mammals these K^+ channel subfamilies are known as Kv1, Kv2, Kv3 and Kv4 channels, respectively.

Voltage-sensitive K^+ channels are homo- or heterotetrameric structures comprised of principal pore-forming alpha-subunits from the same subfamily. Each alpha-subunit has six transmembrane domains, consisting of a voltage sensor at S4 and a pore region at S5–S6. These channels commonly possess a kink in the S6 helices near the activation gate, owing to a Pro-X-Pro sequence, which causes a reduction in the size of a K^+ channel's inner cavity.

Cardiac potassium channels

Cardiac K^+ channels govern a diverse set of important physiological functions, such as heart rate and AP morphology and duration, and they play a pivotal role in regulating cardiac repolarization and establishing the heart's resting state. In terms of voltage-sensitive cardiac K^+ channels, two distinct types exist: transient outward and delayed rectifier channels. However, other voltage-independent cardiac K^+ channels also play a role in repolarization.

Our knowledge and understanding of cardiac K^+ channels has grown substantially in the past 50 years; studies have enabled us to identify different K^+ channel currents and their roles in cardiac repolarization based on their pharmacological and biophysical properties. In addition to this, genetic studies have enabled us to identify the pathological consequences of altered K^+ channel function in response to genetic mutations or drugs which result in QT prolongation. These findings have enabled us to establish links between K^+ channel function and pharmacology in physiological conditions and in disease states.

The transient outward potassium channel

At the very least, the transient outward current (I_{to}) plays an important role in the cardiac AP by controlling Phase 1 of the action potential; a short-lived period of repolarization in between prominent influxes of depolarizing Na^+ and Ca^{2+} ions. However, further examination of this current reveals its crucial role in helping to coordinate complex patterns of repolarization in the heart and from preventing the occurrence of lethal heart rhythm abnormalities.

A number of studies have shown that I_{to} is comprised of two distinct components, I_{to},fast ($I_{to,f}$) and I_{to},slow ($I_{to,s}$). Both $I_{to,f}$ and $I_{to,s}$ are rapidly activating and inactivating, however, they derive their names from differences in the speed in which they recover from steady state inactivation: fast ($I_{to,f}$) and slow ($I_{to,s}$). These current components can also be separated out pharmacologically using Heteropoda toxin-2, which selectively inhibits $I_{to,f}$ at nanomolar (nM) concentrations.

The molecular correlates comprising I_{to} have been shown to be members of the Kv4 and Kv1 K^+ channel families. A mutation in Kv4.2 eliminated $I_{to,f}$ in all ventricular cells from a genetically modified mouse heart (Barry *et al.*, 1998). However, further studies have suggested that in the murine heart, $I_{to,f}$ is comprised of the heteromeric assembly of Kv4.2 and Kv4.3 channels (Guo *et al.*, 2002). In the human heart, due to a lack of expression of Kv4.2, $I_{to,f}$ is thought to be comprised exclusively of Kv4.3 (Dixon *et al.*, 1996). Using a genetically modified mouse heart with a complete knockout of the Kv1.4 gene, Guo *et al.* (1999) demonstrated that $I_{to,s}$ is eliminated in septal cells of Kv1.4 homozygous −/− mice compared to wild-type mice, suggesting that Kv1.4 encodes $I_{to,s}$ in the mouse heart (Guo *et al.*, 1999).

Delayed rectifier potassium channels

Delayed rectifier K^+ currents (I_K) have been extensively studied in canine (Liu and Antzelevitch, 1995), feline (Aiba *et al.*, 2005) and mouse hearts (Babij *et al.*, 1998). Multiple components of I_K can be identified in most hearts based on electrophysiological and pharmacological properties. Two components of I_K based upon differences in activation kinetics, exist in larger mammalian hearts — rapidly activating, I_{Kr}, and slowly activating, I_{Ks}, K^+ channels. In rodent hearts, additional components of I_K have been identified (Nerbonne *et al.*, 2001). Reductions in I_{Kr} and I_{Ks} due to inherited mutations (Jiang *et al.*, 1994; Keating *et al.*, 1991) or unwanted actions of drugs underlie QT prolongation and cardiac arrhythmias.

The ultra rapid delayed rectifier potassium channel

I_{Kur} is a rapidly activating K^+ current and studies have concluded that I_{Kur} inactivates slowly throughout the duration of the AP; the Kv1.5 channel protein constitutes I_{Kur} in larger mammalian hearts (Wang *et al.*, 1993). I_{Kur} has been recorded in human atrial but not ventricular myocytes and selective blockers of Kv1.5 channels may be effective in the treatment of atrial fibrillation (AF) (Knobloch *et al.*, 2002). Rapid atrial pacing has been demonstrated to cause both an immediate and transient increase in Kv1.5 mRNA levels, which could possibly explain the fast reduction in atrial refractoriness observed upon the induction of AF (Yamashita *et al.*, 2000). In this respect, drugs that block I_{Kur} may prevent atrial AP shortening and the onset of AF.

The HERG potassium channel

The HERG K^+ channel, encoded by the human ether-a-go-go related gene (HERG), is thought to be the molecular correlate for I_{Kr}

(Sanguinetti *et al.*, 1995). When I_{Kr} is recorded from ventricular myocytes and from mammalian cells expressing the HERG K^+ channel, distinct gating, external K^+ regulation, and drug sensitivity differences are seen (Clancy *et al.*, 2003). This suggests the presence of an auxiliary modulatory subunit in the native environment. Abbott and colleagues (1999) demonstrated that co-expression of the HERG K^+ channel alongside minK-related protein 1 (MiRP1; encoded by the KCNE2 gene) generates currents closely resembling native I_{Kr} (Abbott *et al.*, 1999).

Class III antiarrhythmic drugs, in particular the methanesulfonanilides group comprising dofetilide and the experimental compound E-4031, have been shown to be potent blockers of the HERG K^+ channel (Clancy *et al.*, 2003; Follmer and Colatsky, 1990). Furthermore over the past decade pharmacological inhibition of HERG K^+ channels has been associated with an increased risk of cardiac arrhythmias. For instance arrhythmias have been reported in up to 1%–5% of patients receiving dofetilide treatment (Mounsey and DiMarco, 2000). As a result of this there has been a reduced interest in the use of HERG K^+ channel inhibitors in antiarrhythmic therapy. Methanesulfonanilides are thought to gain access to the channel pore upon depolarization and bind to a site near the selectivity filter of the channel. However, once inside the channel, these drugs become trapped when the activation gate of the channel closes during repolarization (Mitcheson *et al.*, 2000).

HERG K^+ channels have two key structural features that are considered to underlie the channel's ability to be blocked by an array of drugs that vary in both structure and size. Firstly, HERG K^+ channels lack the PXP motif that is usually found in the S6 helix of Kv1–Kv4 channels. Ordinarily this sequence acts to reduce the size of the channel's inner cavity, thus preventing larger compounds from becoming trapped within the channel. Secondly, the presence of amino acid residues within the S6 region of the channel (Y652 and F656) are believed to interact with many drugs to facilitate their binding to the HERG K^+ channel (Vandenberg *et al.*, 2001).

The slowly activating delayed rectifier potassium channel

The KCNQ1 K^+ channel encodes I_{Ks}, which is a slowly activating K^+ current that plays an important role in atrial and ventricular repolarization. Fast heart rates prevent the complete deactivation of I_{Ks}, resulting in the cumulative build up of I_{Ks} and the subsequent accelerated rate of cardiac repolarization (Faber and Rudy, 2000; Tamargo *et al.*, 2004). Due to the fact that I_{Ks} accumulates at higher heart rates, theoretically, blockers of this component will display greater efficacy at prolonging the cardiac AP at faster rates (Tamargo *et al.*, 2004). A study in ventricular myocytes demonstrated that the selective I_{Ks} blocker chromanol 293B increased the duration of the cardiac AP in a frequency-dependent manner (Bosch *et al.*, 1998). I_{Ks} is formed by the co-assembly of four pore-forming KCNQ1 alpha-subunit proteins alongside two KCNE1 beta-subunit proteins (Chen *et al.*, 2003). Heterologous expression of KCNQ1 in the presence of KCNE1 fully recapitulates the native I_{Ks} current (Sanguinetti *et al.*, 1996).

Inwardly rectifying potassium channels

Inwardly rectifying K^+ channels play an important role in myocardial repolarization. These K^+ currents can be separated out from voltage-sensitive K^- currents on the basis of their channel biophysics: inwardly rectifying K^+ currents are voltage independent, and by their nature they are capable of passing a greater inward as opposed to outward K^+ currents. The outward K^+ current carried by these channels contributes to the later phases of cardiac repolarization and in mediating the heart's electrical resting state. In ventricular myocytes two inwardly rectifying K^+ currents have been described: I_{K1} and I_{KATP}.

The identification of the molecular correlates for I_{K1} was aided by the work of Zaritsky and colleagues (2001) who engineered mice lacking the genes encoding Kir2.1 and Kir2.2 K^+ channel subunits. Whole cell recordings in ventricular myocytes lacking Kir2.1 failed to detect I_{K1} at an extracellular K^+ concentration ($[K^+]_o$) of 4 mM, but detected a very small, residual current at 60 mM $[K^+]_o$ (Zaritsky *et al.*, 2001). Additionally, myocytes lacking Kir2.1 displayed significant APD prolongation (Zaritsky *et al.*, 2001). Myocytes lacking Kir2.2 showed a 50% reduction in I_{K1} suggesting the possibility that both Kir2.1 and Kir2.2 may form functional channels to give rise to I_{K1}. These data suggest that: (1) Kir2.1 is the prominent component of I_{K1} in the mouse heart and (2) that I_{K1} can contribute to AP repolarization.

I_{KATP} is a weakly inwardly rectifying K^+ channel current which is formed by the co-assembly of Kir6.2 and SUR2A subunits: deletion of Kir6.2 eliminates I_{KATP} (Suzuki *et al.*, 2001) and deletion of SUR2 reduces I_{KATP} current density. A decrease in intracellular ATP that occurs in conditions such as hypoxia and ischemia (Noma, 1983) opens these channels, giving rise to an outward current. In this respect these K^+ channels are considered to provide a functional link between the metabolic state of the myocardium and its membrane potential. Additionally, under physiological conditions, pharmacological activation using nicorandil can give rise to a substantial outward current which can shorten cardiac APD (Shimizu and Antzelevitch, 2000).

Species-dependent variability of potassium channels

It is still unclear as to what extent I_{Kr} and I_{Ks} contribute to repolarization in the adult mouse. Developmental studies have shown that I_{Kr} and I_{Ks} are easily detectable and are prominent repolarizing currents in neonatal mouse ventricular myocytes (Wang *et al.*, 1996). However, the densities of I_{Kr} and I_{Ks} have been shown to decrease during postnatal development (Davies *et al.*, 1996). Despite these findings, however, genetically modified mouse hearts with either mutations in or removal of the genes encoding murine I_{Kr} (murine ether-a-go-go related gene, mERG), I_{Ks} (KCNQ1) and the beta-subunit KCNE1 have yielded contrasting results. Mice expressing a mutation in the HERG K^+ channel exhibit prolonged APDs at the single cell level and irregularities in T wave morphology at the whole animal level (Babij *et al.*, 1998). Additionally the mice have delayed repolarization and arrhythmias (London *et al.*, 1998). In wild type (WT) adult murine ventricular myocytes a delayed rectifier current with identical biophysical and pharmacological properties to I_{Kr} recorded in human and guinea pig ventricular myocytes has been consistently reported (Babij *et al.*, 1998; Liu *et al.*, 2004). Pharmacological blockade of I_{Kr} using E-4031 and sotalol prolonged endocardial and epicardial APDs in intact ventricular preparations and at the whole heart level respectively, suggesting the presence of I_{Kr} transmurally in the murine ventricle (Charpentier *et al.*, 1998; Fabritz *et al.*, 2003). In wild type adult mouse ventricular preparations, the selective I_{Ks} blocker chromanol 293B prolonged APD suggesting the presence of I_{Ks} in the wild type adult murine heart (Charpentier *et al.*, 1998). Charpentier *et al.* (1998) reported that deletion of the KCNE1 gene results in a lack of functional I_{Ks} in adult mouse ventricular myocytes, and a lack of sensitivity to chromanol 293B. A complementary study by Drici and colleagues (1998) also suggested that I_{Ks} plays a role in ventricular repolarization in the adult mouse. They reported that mice lacking the KCNE1 subunit display prolonged QT intervals and, at the single cell level, myocytes lack a chromanol 293B-sensitive current (Drici *et al.*, 1998). More recently, experiments performed in genetically modified mouse hearts lacking KCNE1 have documented cardiac arrhythmias (Balasubramaniam *et al.*, 2003).

Potassium channel subunits

At present, a number of auxiliary subunits have been identified for voltage-sensitive K^+ channels, the first being minK (KCNE1), which when co-expressed alongside KCNQ1 forms functional K^+ channels that give rise to I_{Ks} (Barhanin *et al.*, 1996). Genetically engineered mice lacking minK present with inner ear defects, prolonged cardiac APDs and arrhythmias due to a lack of functional I_{Ks} (Balasubramaniam *et al.*, 2003; Drici *et al.*, 1998; Thomas *et al.*, 2007). These findings fully recapitulate the human clinical phenotype in which mutations in minK produce profound bilateral deafness, impaired ventricular repolarization and cardiac arrhythmias as described by the Jervell and Lange-Nielsen (JLN) Syndrome (Schulze-Bahr *et al.*, 1997). Following the discovery of minK, homologues — minK related peptides (MiRPs) — were identified and it was subsequently shown that MiRP1 (KCNE2) forms a complex with HERG, which fully recapitulates native I_{Kr} (Abbott *et al.*, 1999; Vandenberg *et al.*, 2001).

Accessory proteins for transient outward K$^+$ channels were discovered in the rat brain (An *et al.*, 2000). Of the three proteins identified, termed K$^+$ Channel Interacting Proteins (KChIPs), KChIP2 is expressed in the heart. KChIPs are small proteins that considerably increase the magnitude of I_{to} (by over eight times) when co-expressed with K$^+$ channels in cells by enhancing K$^+$ channel trafficking to the plasma membrane. Kuo and colleagues (2001) engineered mice lacking KChIP2 to study the role of these accessory subunits in regulating cardiac repolarization: deletion of KChIP2 significantly increased repolarization times.

Summary

Cardiac myocytes express a broad range of ion channels with discrete voltage- and time- dependent properties. Alterations in the properties of these ion channels, due to drugs or disease, can profoundly disrupt the heart's electrical properties, causing electrical instability and the generation of potentially lethal ventricular arrhythmias. The following chapters examine a number of human clinical arrhythmia disorders that stem from dysfunctional cardiac ion channels and describe the mechanisms underlying cardiac arrhythmias.

References

Abbott, G.W. *et al.* (1999). MiRP1 forms IKr potassium channels with HERG and is associated with cardiac arrhythmia. *Cell*, **97**, 175–187.

Aiba, T. *et al.* (2005). Cellular and ionic mechanism for drug-induced long QT syndrome and effectiveness of verapamil. *J Am Coll Cardiol*, **45**, 300–307.

An, W.F. *et al.* (2000). Modulation of A-type potassium channels by a family of calcium sensors. *Nature,* **403,** 553–556.

Anderson, M.E. (2004). Calmodulin kinase and L-type calcium channels; a recipe for arrhythmias? *Trends Cardiovasc Med,* **14,** 152–161.

Babij, P. *et al.* (1998). Inhibition of cardiac delayed rectifier K^+ current by overexpression of the long-QT syndrome HERG G628S mutation in transgenic mice. *Circ Res,* **83,** 668–678.

Balasubramaniam, R. *et al.* (2003). Electrogram prolongation and nifedipine-suppressible ventricular arrhythmias in mice following targeted disruption of KCNE1. *J Physiol,* **552,** 535–546.

Bangalore, R. *et al.* (1996). Influence of L-type Ca channel alpha 2/delta-subunit on ionic and gating current in transiently transfected HEK 293 cells. *Am J Physiol,* **270,** H1521–1528.

Barhanin, J. *et al.* (1996). K(V)LQT1 and IsK (minK) proteins associate to form the I(Ks) cardiac potassium current. *Nature,* **384,** 78–80.

Barry, D.M. *et al.* (1998). Functional knockout of the transient outward current, long-QT syndrome, and cardiac remodeling in mice expressing a dominant-negative Kv4 alpha subunit. *Circ Res,* **83,** 560–567.

Bosch, R.F. *et al.* (1998). Effects of the chromanol 293B, a selective blocker of the slow, component of the delayed rectifier K^+ current, on repolarization in human and guinea pig ventricular myocytes. *Cardiovasc Res,* **38,** 441–450.

Charpentier, F. *et al.* (1998). Adult KCNE1-knockout mice exhibit a mild cardiac cellular phenotype. *Biochem Biophys Res Commun,* **251,** 806–810.

Chen, H. *et al.* (2003). Charybdotoxin binding in the I(Ks) pore demonstrates two MinK subunits in each channel complex. *Neuron,* **40,** 15–23.

Clancy, C.E., *et al.* (2003). K^+ channel structure-activity relationships and mechanisms of drug-induced QT prolongation. *Annu Rev Pharmacol Toxicol,* **43,** 441–461.

Davies, M.P. *et al.* (1996). Developmental changes in ionic channel activity in the embryonic murine heart. *Circ Res,* **78,** 15–25.

Dixon, J.E. *et al.* (1996). Role of the Kv4.3 K^+ channel in ventricular muscle. A molecular correlate for the transient outward current. *Circ Res,* **79,** 659–668.

Drici, M.D. *et al.* (1998). Involvement of IsK-associated K^+ channel in heart rate control of repolarization in a murine engineered model of Jervell and Lange-Nielsen syndrome. *Circ Res,* **83,** 95–102.

Faber, G.M. and Rudy, Y. (2000). Action potential and contractility changes in [Na($^+$)](i) overloaded cardiac myocytes: a simulation study. *Biophys J*, **78**, 2392–2404.

Fabiato, A. and Fabiato, F. (1972). Excitation-contraction coupling of isolated cardiac fibers with disrupted or closed sarcolemmas. Calcium-dependent cyclic and tonic contractions. *Circ Res*, **31**, 293–307.

Fabritz, L. *et al.* (2003). Prolonged action potential durations, increased dispersion of repolarization, and polymorphic ventricular tachycardia in a mouse model of proarrhythmia. *Basic Res Cardiol*, **98**, 25–32.

Follmer, C.H. and Colatsky, T.J. (1990). Block of delayed rectifier potassium current, IK, by flecainide and E-4031 in cat ventricular myocytes. *Circulation*, **82**, 289–293.

Guo, W. *et al.* (2002). Role of heteromultimers in the generation of myocardial transient outward K+ currents. *Circ Res*, **90**, 586–593.

Guo, W. *et al.* (1999). Molecular basis of transient outward K$^+$ current diversity in mouse ventricular myocytes. *J Physiol*, **521**, 587–599.

Jiang, C. *et al.* (1994). Two long QT syndrome loci map to chromosomes 3 and 7 with evidence for further heterogeneity. *Nat Genet*, **8**, 141–147.

Keating, M. *et al.* (1991). Linkage of a cardiac arrhythmia, the long QT syndrome, and the Harvey ras-1 gene. *Science*, **252**, 704–706.

Knobloch, K. *et al.* (2002). Electrophysiological and antiarrhythmic effects of the novel I(Kur) channel blockers, S9947 and S20951, on left vs. right pig atrium *in vivo* in comparison with the I(Kr) blockers dofetilide, azimilide, d,l-sotalol and ibutilide. *Naunyn Schmiedebergs Arch Pharmacol*, **366**, 482–487.

Kuo, H.C. *et al.* (2001). A defect in the Kv channel-interacting protein 2 (KChIP2) gene leads to a complete loss of I(to) and confers susceptibility to ventricular tachycardia. *Cell*, **107**, 801–813.

Liu, D.W. and Antzelevitch, C. (1995). Characteristics of the delayed rectifier current (IKr and IKs) in canine ventricular epicardial, midmyocardial, and endocardial myocytes. A weaker IKs contributes to the longer action potential of the M cell. *Circ Res*, **76**, 351–365.

Liu, G.X. *et al.* (2004). Single-channel recordings of a rapid delayed rectifier current in adult mouse ventricular myocytes: basic properties and effects of divalent cations. *J Physiol*, **556**, 401–413.

London, B. *et al.* (1998). QT interval prolongation and arrhythmias in heterozygous Merg1-targeted mice (abstract). *Circulation*, 98, I–56.

Mitcheson, J.S. *et al.* (2000). A structural basis for drug-induced long QT syndrome. *Proc Natl Acad Sci USA*, 97, 12329–12333.

Mounsey, J.P. and DiMarco, J.P. (2000). Cardiovascular drugs. Dofetilide. *Circulation*, 102, 2665–2670.

Nerbonne, J.M. *et al.* (2001). Genetic manipulation of cardiac K($^+$) channel function in mice: what have we learned, and where do we go from here? *Circ Res*, 89, 944–956.

Noma, A. (1983). ATP-regulated K$^+$ channels in cardiac muscle. *Nature*, 305, 147–148.

Sanguinetti, M.C. *et al.* (1996). Coassembly of K(V)LQT1 and minK (IsK) proteins to form cardiac I(Ks) potassium channel. *Nature*, 384, 80–83.

Sanguinetti, M.C. *et al.* (1995). A mechanistic link between an inherited and an acquired cardiac arrhythmia: HERG encodes the IKr potassium channel. *Cell*, 81, 299–307.

Schulze-Bahr, E. *et al.* (1997). KCNE1 mutations cause jervell and Lange-Nielsen syndrome. *Nat Genet*, 17, 267–268.

Shimizu, W. and Antzelevitch, C. (2000). Effects of a K($^+$) channel opener to reduce transmural dispersion of repolarization and prevent torsade de pointes in LQT1, LQT2, and LQT3 models of the long-QT syndrome. *Circulation*, 102, 706–712.

Suzuki, M. *et al.* (2001). Functional roles of cardiac and vascular ATP-sensitive potassium channels clarified by Kir6.2-knockout mice. *Circ Res*, 88, 570–577.

Tamargo, J. *et al.* (2004). Pharmacology of cardiac potassium channels. *Cardiovasc Res*, 62, 9–33.

Thomas, G. *et al.* (2007). Mechanisms of ventricular arrhythmogenesis in mice following targeted disruption of KCNE1 modelling long QT 5 syndrome. *J Physiol*, 578, 99–114.

Vandenberg, J.I. *et al.* (2001). HERG K$^+$ channels: friend and foe. *Trends Pharmacol Sci*, 22, 240–246.

Wang, L. *et al.* (1996). Developmental changes in the delayed rectifier K$^+$ channels in mouse heart. *Circ Res*, 79, 79–85.

Wang, Z. *et al.* (1993). Sustained depolarization-induced outward current in human atrial myocytes. Evidence for a novel delayed rectifier K+ current similar to Kv1.5 cloned channel currents. *Circ Res,* **73**, 1061–1076.

Wu, Y. *et al.* (2002). Calmodulin kinase II and arrhythmias in a mouse model of cardiac hypertrophy. *Circulation,* **106**, 1288–1293.

Yamaguchi, H. *et al.* (1998). Multiple modulation pathways of calcium channel activity by a beta subunit. Direct evidence of beta subunit participation in membrane trafficking of the alpha1C subunit. *J Biol Chem,* **273**, 19348–19356.

Yamashita, T. *et al.* (2000). Short-term effects of rapid pacing on mRNA level of voltage-dependent K(+) channels in rat atrium: electrical remodeling in paroxysmal atrial tachycardia. *Circulation,* **101**, 2007–2014.

Zaritsky, J.J. *et al.* (2001). The consequences of disrupting cardiac inwardly rectifying K(+) current (I(K1)) as revealed by the targeted deletion of the murine Kir2.1 and Kir2.2 genes. *J Physiol,* **533**, 697–710.

CHAPTER 3

Clinical Arrhythmia Syndromes

Introduction

Cardiac myocytes express a wide array of ion channels that govern the heart's ability to contract and pump blood throughout the body. Dysfunctions in cardiac ion channels, due to disease or drugs, can cause the heart to become electrically unstable and lead to the generation of abnormal cardiac rhythms (arrhythmias) and sudden death. The purpose of this chapter is to provide a succinct overview of several of the most defining clinical features of congenital Long QT Syndrome (LQTS) and drug-induced QT prolongation and proarrhythmia. In particular, this chapter examines several important cases of drug-induced proarrhythmia that have resulted in the withdrawal of drugs from major pharmaceutical markets.

The Long QT Syndrome

The measurement of the QT interval on the ECG, reflecting the time taken for complete ventricular repolarization following depolarization, is one of the simplest and most frequently used methods for the clinical assessment of repolarization. The Long QT Syndrome is a collection of primary electrical disorders of the heart that are characterized by a prolonged QT interval (this equates to a QT interval greater than 440 ms or 460 ms in males and females, respectively) and an increased risk of ventricular arrhythmias and sudden cardiac death. As discussed in Chapter 2, the QT interval is a marker of the ventricular action potential duration (APD); a prolonged QT interval signals impaired repolarization which may result from reduced levels of outward repolarizing K^+ currents or increased levels of inward, depolarizing ionic currents. The pathological changes to cardiac ion channel function seen in LQTS may result from inheritable forms of LQTS (congenital LQTS), where mutations can alter the function of ion channels, or due to the effects of drugs on ion channels, which is known as drug-induced QT prolongation (acquired LQTS).

A prolongation of the QT interval dramatically increases the risk of developing potentially lethal ventricular arrhythmias, and one particular arrhythmia, Torsade de Pointes (TdP), has been commonly associated with a prolonged QT interval. The term TdP was coined to describe a rapid, polymorphic ventricular arrhythmia that was first seen in a female patient with heart block in which the QRS complexes of the ECG appeared to repeatedly twist around the isoelectric line. TdP has since become one of the most commonly used terms to describe a polymorphic ventricular tachycardia in the setting of a prolonged QT interval. The onset of TdP has typically been found to follow a similar pattern in which depolarizations measured on the ECG occur in a short-long-short sequence; after an initial premature ventricular depolarization, a compensatory pause takes place followed by another premature ventricular depolarization, occurring within the T wave, which initiates the arrhythmia (TdP, and its common pattern of onset, is illustrated in Figure 1). Importantly, TdP may degenerate into the far more lethal arrhythmia, ventricular fibrillation, which may rapidly lead to syncope and death within minutes of onset.

Congenital Long QT Syndrome

Correlations between QT prolongation and sudden cardiac death (SCD) originate from early descriptions of congenital arrhythmia syndromes associated with prolonged QT intervals (Jervell and Lange-Nielsen, 1957; Romano *et al.*, 1963; Ward, 1964). The first

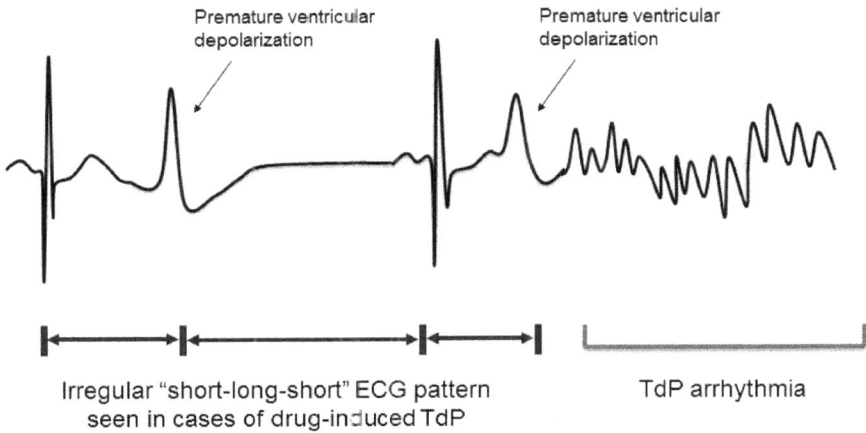

Figure 1: An example of an ECG trace of drug-induced QT prolongation and Torsade de Pointes arrhythmia.

report of SCD due to congenital LQTS may date back to the mid-19th century when a clinical report described the case of a young female with congenital deafness, "who collapsed and died while being publicly admonished at school." It later became clear that two of the female's siblings had also suddenly died, "after a terrible fright and a violent fit of rage," (Meissner, 1856). Almost a century later, in 1953, a clinical report described a patient who developed multiple episodes of a polymorphic ventricular arrhythmia, resembling TdP, in the setting of QT prolongation (Dupler, 1953).

Over 12 different forms of congenital LQTS, representing a range of mutations in different cardiac ion channels, have so far been described; however, mutations in the Na^+ channel, and the KCNQ1 and HERG K^+ channels account for almost 75% of documented cases of congenital LQTS. The vast majority (two-thirds) of congenital LQTS cases result from loss-of-function mutations in the KCNQ1 (LQT 1 Syndrome) and HERG (LQT 2 Syndrome) K^+ channels which impair repolarization and prolong the QT interval.

Gain-of-function mutations in the Na^+ channel (LQT 3 Syndrome), in which a persistent, depolarizing Na^+ current impedes repolarization and induces QT prolongation, are considered to account for approximately 5%–10% of congenital LQTS cases (Drew *et al.*, 2010). Clinically, LQT 3 Syndrome differs from other forms of congenital LQTS in many aspects; in LQT 3 Syndrome fatal arrhythmias occur in 39% of patients during sleep or rest but in LQT 1 and LQT 2 Syndromes, lethal arrhythmias are associated with stress or arousal (Schwartz *et al.*, 2001).

Extensive research into congenital forms of LQTS has led to a much greater understanding of the risks of arrhythmia due to QT prolongation. Based on studies of congenital LQTS, it appears that arrhythmia risk is associated with the degree of QT prolongation; the greater the QT prolongation, the greater the risk of developing TdP — each 10 ms increase in the QT interval has been proposed to result in a 5%–7% exponential increased risk of TdP in congenital LQTS patients (Moss *et al.*, 1991; Zareba *et al.*, 1998). Additionally, congenital LQTS patients have almost a three-fold higher risk of TdP if they present with a QT interval exceeding 500 ms (Priori *et al.*, 2003; Sauer *et al.*, 2007).

Drug-Induced QT Prolongation

The potential for a wide range of drugs, both cardiovascular and non-cardiovascular, to prolong the QT interval and induce potentially lethal ventricular arrhythmias is currently one of the greatest challenges facing drug developers. Today, well over 200 different medications have been associated with drug-induced proarrhythmia, according to the World Health Organization's Drug Monitoring Centre (Darpo, 2001) and this major adverse event has led to the withdrawal or restricted use of a large number of medications covering a range of indications. Risk factors for drug-induced QT prolongation and TdP are listed in Table 1, and potential treatment algorithms for patients presenting with QT prolongation and proarrhythmia are depicted in Figures 2 and 3.

Several lines of evidence suggest that patients who develop drug-induced QT prolongation possess an underlying genetic predisposition to TdP. Clinical studies of congenital LQTS have recognized the

Table 1:   Risk Factors for Drug-Induced Arrhythmias.

Risk Factor
QT prolongation or other repolarization abnormalities at baseline
Cardiovascular disease (heart failure, myocardial infarction, cardiomyopathy)
Electrolyte abnormalities (hypokalemia, hypomagnesemia, hypocalcemia)
The use of diuretic therapy (diuretics can increase the risk of hypokalemia)
Bradycardia
Reduced ability to metabolize drugs (either due to drugs inhibiting key hepatic enzymes or through disease)
Subclinical forms of repolarization abnormalities
Female sex

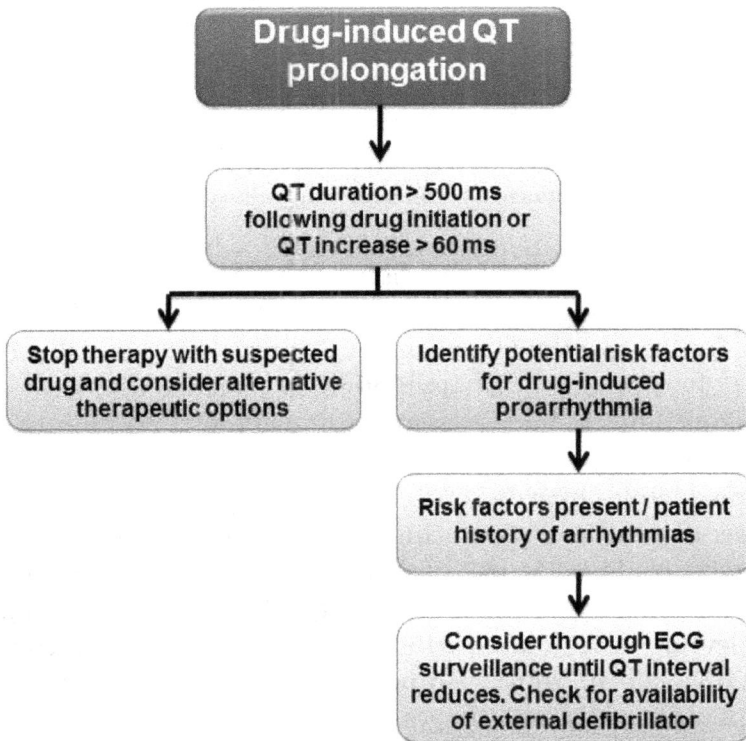

Figure 2:   Potential treatment algorithm for drug-induced QT prolongation.

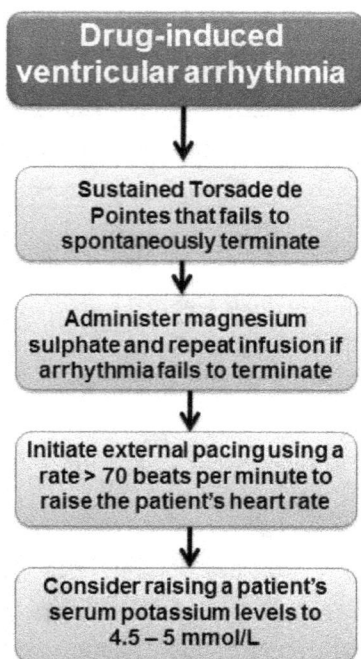

Figure 3:   Potential treatment algorithm for drug-induced ventricular arrhythmias.

incomplete penetrance of the disease (Priori *et al.*, 1999). Vincent *et al.* (1992) highlighted the fact that 6% of gene carriers from three LQT1 families possessed a normal QT interval. Additionally, Priori *et al.* (1999) proposed that asymptomatic patients, who have LQTS mutations but do not present with overt QT prolongation or arrhythmias, may exist in cases where only one family member has presented clinically with LQTS. These findings indicate that a large number of patients with subclinical mutations in cardiac ion channels, who could be at risk of drug-induced QT prolongation and proarrhythmia, exist. Indeed, it is thought that 5% to 10% of patients who develop drug-induced TdP have a subclinical form of congenital LQTS (Roden, 2004). Furthermore, the QT interval measured at baseline is frequently longer in patients who go on to develop drug-induced QT prolongation than those who tolerate the drug well (Sesti *et al.*, 2000).

The Arizona Centre for Education and Research on Therapeutics (CERT) maintains lists of drugs that have a potential risk of QT prolongation and proarrhythmia; almost 100 drugs are listed and almost a third of these are generally accepted by the institute's advisory board as having a risk of inducing TdP. Of the remaining drugs listed by the Arizona CERT, 47 are described as having a possible risk of inducing TdP (drugs that induce QT prolongation and/or have been associated with TdP but substantial evidence demonstrating proarrhythmia is lacking) and 23 have a conditional risk of TdP (drugs with a risk of QT prolongation and/or proarrhythmia only under certain conditions).

As illustrated in Figure 4, approximately 30% (nine) of these drugs are cardiovascular therapeutics, seven of which are antiarrhythmic drugs. These findings are unsurprising given the intentional, direct effects of antiarrhythmic drugs on cardiac ion channels and the patient populations to which they are prescribed. The risk of QT prolongation and proarrhythmia with quinidine (a Class IA antiarrhythmic) is well known; arrhythmias have been estimated to occur in up to 8% of quinidine-treated patients (Cramer *et al.*, 1968;

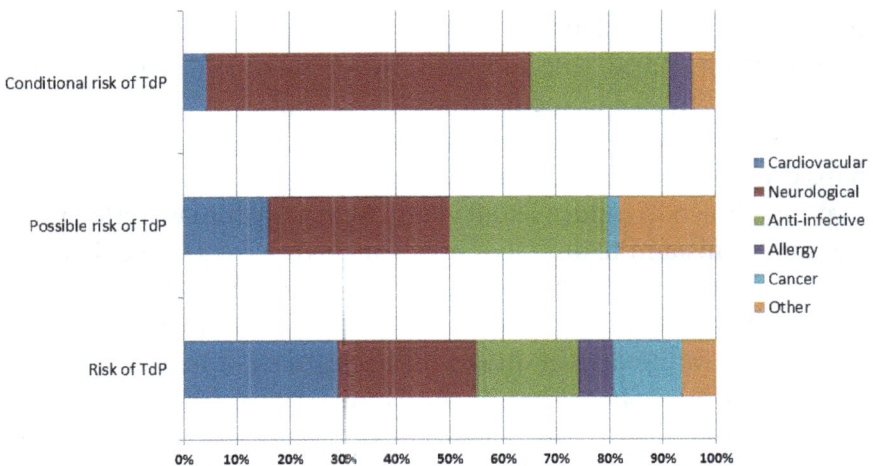

Figure 4: **Drugs, categorized by therapeutic sector, that are associated with different levels of risk of proarrhythmia.**

Radford *et al.*, 1968; Roden *et al.*, 1986). Indeed, perhaps one of the earliest reports of drug-induced QT prolongation and proarrhythmia dates back to the 1920s with a description of multiple episodes of syncope occurring in a patient receiving quinidine therapy (Roden, 2004).

Sotalol (a Class III antiarrhythmic) has also been associated with proarrhythmia; according to the drug's prescribing information, in clinical trials of sotalol, involving over 3000 patients with cardiac arrhythmias, TdP occurred in approximately 4% of high risk patients. Owing to the risk of QT prolongation and proarrhythmia with sotalol, patients initiating or reinitiating sotalol therapy are recommended to be placed, for at least three days, in a facility that can provide continuous ECG monitoring and cardiac resuscitation. Dofetilide, another Class III antiarrhythmic has a similar risk of TdP; according to the drug's prescribing information, TdP was reported in 0.8% of patients with supraventricular arrhythmias and in 3.3% of patients with congestive heart failure. Patients initiated on dofetilide therapy must also undergo ECG monitoring for at least three days.

Of perhaps greater concern have been well-documented cases of QT prolongation and arrhythmias induced by non-cardiovascular drugs, including drugs for the treatment of cancer, neurological disorders, allergies, and infections. Of the drugs associated with QT prolongation and/or TdP, and listed by the Arizona CERT, over 81% are non-cardiovascular medications.

Terfenadine-induced QT prolongation and proarrhythmia is perhaps one of the most well-known cases of a non-cardiovascular drug that was shown to induce lethal ventricular arrhythmias. Terfenadine was an antihistamine drug that was launched in the United States in 1985 and heavily used; in 1988 almost 13 million prescriptions for terfenadine were written and by 1998, the year in which it was removed from the market due to cardiac toxicity, it had become the tenth most prescribed drug in the United States (Monahan *et al.*, 1990; Fermini *et al.*, 2003). Initial cases documenting cardiac toxicity with terfenadine were attributed to overdoses with the drug; however, in 1990 the first clinical case of proarrhythmia with therapeutic doses of terfenadine was reported (Monahan *et al.*, 1990). In this report, TdP occurred in a patient receiving terfenadine and keto-conazole; ketoconazole is known to inhibit the CYP-450 drug metabolizing enzymes and it therefore prevented the metabolism and removal of terfenadine, causing the drug to reach toxic concentrations in the body, block HERG K^+ channels, and induce QT prolongation and arrhythmias. Between 1985 and 1996, terfenadine was associated with over 400 major adverse cardiac events, including 98 deaths (Linquist *et al.*, 1997). Following terfenadine's removal from the market the drug was replaced by its metabolite, fexofena-dine, which retained terfenadine's therapeutic effects but lacked its adverse effects on the heart.

Cisapride is another major example of a non-cardiovascular drug linked to QT prolongation and proarrhythmia that was also with-drawn from the market. Cisapride was a prokinetic gastrointestinal drug used for the management of gastroesophageal reflux disease; the drug was launched in the United States in 1993, and by 1996 it was among the top 100 most prescribed medications in the United States with over five million prescriptions annually (Rampe *et al.*, 1997). However, following several case reports of major cardiac tox-icity, cisapride was withdrawn from the market in 2000. Following the drug's removal, a 2001 report detailed the incidence of major car-diac adverse events in patients receiving cisapride (Wysowski *et al.*, 2001). In total the FDA received reports of cardiac toxicity in 341 patients; there were 107 cases of TdP, 25 cases of cardiac arrest, and 15 instances of sudden death (Wysowski *et al.*, 2001). QT prolonga-tion was also seen in 34% of reported cases. In keeping with other drugs associated with QT prolongation and proarrhythmia, cellular studies revealed that cisapride was a potent inhibitor of the HERG K^+ channel (Rampe *et al.*, 1997).

The macrolide antibiotics, in particular erythromycin, have also been implicated in drug-induced QT prolongation and TdP. A report which examined the FDA's Adverse Event Reporting System for cases of TdP associated with macrolide antibiotics effectively illustrated several of the most important risk factors for drug-induced QT pro-longation and proarrhythmia (Shaffer *et al.*, 2002). In total the report identified 156 cases of TdP associated with the use of a macrolide antibiotic. Half of the events were associated solely with the use of a macrolide and no other drug capable of prolonging the QT interval, whereas the remaining 78 reports of TdP occurred in patients who were also receiving a QT-prolonging drug, the most common of which was cisapride (Shaffer *et al.*, 2002). On average TdP events were reported just four to nine days after starting macrolide therapy and patients' QT intervals were significantly prolonged when TdP was documented, compared to baseline measurements (594 ms vs. 432 ms, respectively). Patients developing TdP also commonly had a pre-existing cardiovascular condition; 42% of patients had at least one cardiac disorder — the two most conditions were cardiomyopathy and heart failure, which were found in 23% and 24% of all TdP cases, respectively. Other major risk factors for drug-induced QT prolongation and proarrhythmia were also found among the TdP cases. Hypokalemia and hypomagnesemia, for example, were reported in 17% and 21% of cases, respectively (Shaffer *et al.*, 2002). These findings with erythromycin highlight several important risk factors that can contribute to proarrhythmia with QT-prolonging drugs: cardiovascular comorbidities and electrolyte abnormalities.

Summary

Based on clinical studies of congenital LQTS patients, increases in the QT interval appears to increase the risk of developing ventricular arrhythmias, particularly TdP which may degenerate into VF. Drug-induced QT prolongation and proarrhythmia is a complex, major adverse event associated with many different drugs and risk factors. Over 200 drugs have been implicated in prolonging the QT interval and increasing the risk of proarrhythmia; in particular, antiarrhythmic drugs appear to carry the greatest risk of inducing arrhythmias in patients. Arrhythmias and sudden death linked to terfenadine and cisapride are two of the most prominent cases of proarrhythmia leading to drug withdrawals. The next chapter examines the mechanisms that are responsible for the initiation of arrhythmias.

References

Cramer, G. (1968). Early and late results of conversion of atrial fibrillation with quinidine. A clinical and hemodynamic study. *Acta Med Scand Suppl*, **490**, 5–102.

Darpo, B. (2001). Spectrum of drugs prolonging the QT interval and the incidence of torsades de pointes. *Eur Heart J Suppl*, **3**, K70–K80.

Drew, B. *et al.* (2010). Prevention of torsade de pointes in hospital settings: a scientific statement from the American Heart Association and the American College of Cardiology Foundation. *Circulation*, **121**, 1047–1060.

Dupler, D. (1953). Ventricular arrhythmia and Stokes-Adams syndrome. *Circulation*, **7**, 585.

Fermini, B. *et al.* (2003). The impact of drug-induced QT interval prolongation on drug discovery and development. *Nat Rev Drug Discov*, **2**, 439–447.

Jervell, A. and Lange-Nielsen, F. (1957). Congenital deaf-mutism, functional heart disease with prolongation of the Q-T interval and sudden death. *Am Heart J*, **54**, 59–68.

Linquist, M. *et al.* (1997). Risks of non-sedating antihistamines. *Lancet*, **349**, 1322.

Meissner, F.L. (1856). Taubstummheit und Taubstummenbildung. *Leipzig and Heidelberg*, 119–120.

Monahan, B. *et al.* (1990). Torsades de Pointes occurring in association with terfenadine use. *JAMA*, **264**, 2788–2790.

Moss, A. *et al.* (1991). The long QT syndrome: prospective longitudinal study of 328 families. *Circulation*, **84**, 1136–1144.

Priori, S. *et al.* (1999). Low penetrance in the long-QT syndrome: clinical impact. *Circulation*, **99**, 529–533.

Priori, S. *et al.* (2003). Risk stratification in the long-QT syndrome. *N Engl J Med*, **348**, 1866–1874.

Radford, M. *et al.* (1968). Long-term results of DC reversion of atrial fibrillation. *Br Heart J*, **30**, 91–96.

Rampe, D. *et al.* (1997). A mechanism for the proarrhythmic effects of cisapride (Propulsid): high affinity blockade of the human cardiac potassium channel HERG. *FEBS Lett*, **417**, 28–32.

Roden, D. *et al.* (1986). Incidence and clinical features of the quinidine-associated long QT syndrome: implications for patient care. *Am Heart J*, **111**, 1088–1093.

Roden, D. (2004). Drug-induced prolongation of the QT interval. *N Engl J Med*, **350**, 1013–1022.

Romano, C. *et al.* (1963). [Rare cardiac arrhythmias of the pediatric age. I. Repetitive paroxysmal tachycardia.]. *Minerva Pediatr*, **15**, 1155–1164.

Sauer, A. *et al.* (2007). Long QT syndrome in adults. *J Am Coll Cardiol*, **49**, 329–337.

Schwartz, P. *et al.* (2001). Genotype-phenotype correlation in the long-QT syndrome: gene-specific triggers for life-threatening arrhythmias. *Circulation*, **103**, 89–95.

Sesti, F. *et al.* (2000). A common polymorphism associated with antibiotic-induced cardiac arrhythmia. *Proc Natl Acad Sci USA*, **97**, 10613–10618.

Shaffer, D. *et al.* (2002). Concomitant risk factors in reports of torsade de pointes associated with macrolide use: review of the United States Food and Drug Administration Adverse Event Reporting System. *Clin Infect Dis*, **35**, 197–200.

Vincent, G. *et al.* (1992). The spectrum of symptoms and QT intervals in carriers of the gene for the long-QT syndrome. *N Engl J Med*, **327**, 846–852.

Ward, O.C. (1964). A new familial cardiac syndrome in children. *J Ir Med Assoc*, **54**, 103–106.

Wysowski, D. *et al.* (2001). Postmarketing reports of QT prolongation and ventricular arrhythmia in association with cisapride and Food and Drug Administration regulatory actions. *Am J Gastroenterol*, **96**, 1698–1703.

Zareba, W. *et al.* (1998). Influence of genotype on the clinical course of the long-QT syndrome: International Long-QT Syndrome Registry Research Group. *New Engl J Med*, **339**, 960–965.

CHAPTER 4

The Mechanisms Underlying Cardiac Arrhythmias

Introduction

Despite the high prevalence and societal impact of cardiac arrhythmias, our understanding of the cellular and molecular mechanisms governing the initiation, maintenance and propagation of arrhythmias is still limited. Sudden cardiac death (SCD) resulting from ventricular arrhythmias still poses a major medical challenge and a significant public health burden. Cardiac arrhythmias are one of the most important causes of morbidity and mortality in the developed world and account for over 300,000 deaths per year in the United States (Kannel *et al.*, 1987; Willich *et al.*, 1987) and up to 70,000 deaths per year in the U.K. (NICE, 2000). By focussing on pivotal experimental studies performed over the last 40 years, this chapter explores some of the major mechanisms that are considered to underlie cardiac arrhythmias.

Mechanisms Underlying Cardiac Arrhythmias

The experimental study of arrhythmogenesis dates back to the pivotal findings reported by Mines at the turn of the last century. In a series of elegant papers, Mines proposed the existence of circus movement re-entry as an important mechanism by which arrhythmias can self perpetuate (Mines, 1913). Electrophysiological studies in a variety of model systems, including human hearts, have shed important light on the mechanisms underlying arrhythmias and sudden death in the setting of QT prolongation. Classically, three mechanisms appear to preside over the induction of ventricular arrhythmias: (1) abnormal automaticity; (2) triggered activity; and (3) re-entry.

Abnormal Automaticity

Automaticity, a property of specialized cells within the SA node, establishes a regular coordinated cardiac rhythm. Although the SA node is the main impulse generator in the heart, other regions such as the AV node and Purkinje fibers are capable of generating APs in conditions where SA node function becomes compromised, for example in sick sinus syndrome (Benson *et al.*, 2003). At the clinical level, abnormal automaticity may arise in conditions such as ischemia or infarction, and it has been observed experimentally in Purkinje fibers. Roden and Hoffman (1985) demonstrated that canine Purkinje fibers developed abnormal automaticity at slow pacing rates in the presence of quinidine and hypokalemia (Roden and Hoffman, 1985).

Early and Delayed Afterdepolarizations

Afterdepolarizations are oscillations of a cell's membrane potential that are a function of the preceding action potential (AP). Of particular concern is their ability to generate premature APs (known as triggered beats) if they have a sufficiently high amplitude. Afterdepolarizations can be further subdivided into two separate categories depending on when they occur in the AP: early or delayed afterdepolarizations (EADs and DADs, repectively).

EADs interrupt the smooth repolarization phase of the cardiac AP and they have been recorded during phases 2 or 3 (Figure 1). Experimentally, EADs have been recorded in preparations exposed to drugs implicated in acquired LQTS and in genetically modified hearts modeling human cardiac diseases. A characteristic feature of

Early afterdepolarizations (EADs)   Delayed afterdepolarizations (DADs)

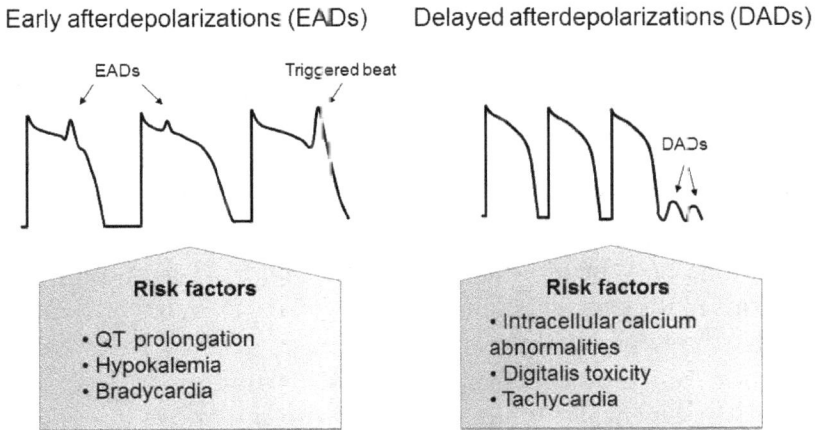

Figure 1: A comparison between the features and risk factors of early and delayed afterdepolarizations.

EADs is their strong rate dependence. A pathologically slow heart rate (known as bradycardia) or a slow artificial pacing rate used in laboratory experiments is often, but not always, necessary for EAD induction. Slow pacing in canine Purkinje fibers or AV node ablation in the isolated heart readily induces EADs and triggered activity: rapid pacing has been shown to suppress these abnormalities.

Several studies have attempted to identify the cellular mechanisms underlying EADs. One of the most widely accepted theories states that EAD induction requires both prolongation of the AP and a recovery from inactivation of the L-type Ca^{2+} channel. When repolarization is impaired, cardiac myocytes spend more time in the depolarized state, where Ca^{2+} channels can open for a second time, permitting another influx of depolarizing Ca^{2+} ions into the cell. A number of other ionic currents, however, have also been proposed as candidates for EADs.

DADs, on the other hand, are oscillations that occur after full repolarization has taken place. In contrast to EADs, DADs are typically associated with rapid heart rates and similar to their earlier counterparts, they too can elicit a premature AP if they reach sufficient amplitudes (Figure 1). DADs are often encountered under conditions of disrupted intracellular Ca^{2+} handling, for example following treatment with cardiac glycosides (drugs commonly used in end-stage heart failure to increase the pumping capability of the heart) or catecholamines. Catecholaminergic polymorphic ventricular tachycardia (CPVT) is an inherited condition that predisposes its sufferers to stress-induced (associated with high heart rates) lethal arrhythmias and SCD. It has now been established that congenital gain-of-function mutations in the gene encoding RyR2 underlie CPVT, in which mutant RyR2 channels permit excessive amounts of Ca^{2+} to leave the sarcoplasmic reticulum. DADs and lethal arrhythmias have been recorded in genetically engineered mice with mutations in RyR2 and subjected to exercise. Ion currents implicated in the generation of DADs include the Na^+-Ca^{2+} exchanger and the Ca^{2+}-activated chloride currents.

Re-entry

Re-entry, a major arrhythmia mechanism, was identified following pioneering work conducted by Mines (Mines, 1913). Following this report a re-entry mechanism, occurring within a theoretical model comprising two branches of a Purkinje bundle, both connected to a section of ventricular tissue, was proposed. According to this model (illustrated in Figure 2), the following series of events would lead to development of a re-entry circuit which could sustain an arrhythmia: (1) an impulse arriving from point A reaches the two Purkinje branches, B and C; (2) branch B is damaged and the electrical impulse cannot travel through the fiber in this direction, but it passes readily along fiber C, and it subsequently stimulates the ventricular muscle at D; (3) the advancing impulse propagates along the ventricular muscle and enters the Purkinje system at E where it would travel through the damaged branch of the Purkinje fiber at a such slow speed as to reach point B when the tissue is no longer refractory and it has recovered from the initial excitation. The re-excitable tissue at point C is once again excited by the late arriving impulse which therefore establishes a re-entrant arrhythmia circuit.

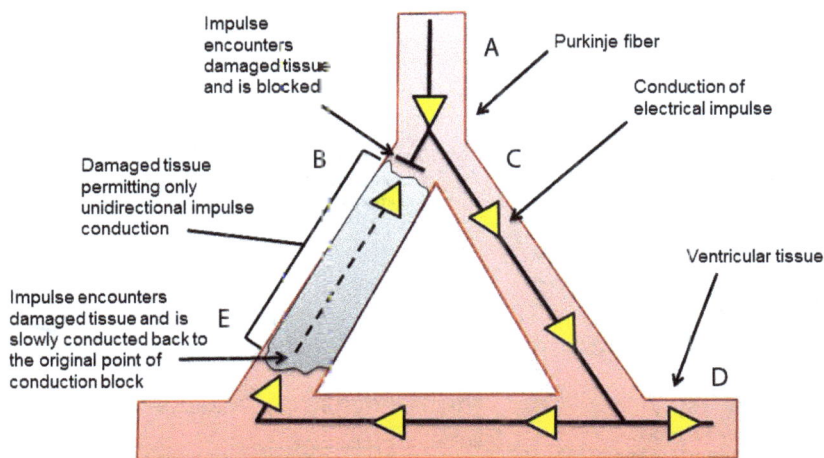

Figure 2: The classical model of arrhythmogenic re-entry.

Whereas the chain of events described above requires the presence of a physical obstacle (in this case, damaged tissue that can only conduct an impulse in one direction) in order to create an arrhythmia circuit, a great deal of work has demonstrated that re-entry can occur in the absence of any physical obstacles; functional re-entry can arise due to regional differences in the heart's electrophysiological profile. Such an example of functional re-entry, the "Leading Circle Model," is illustrated in Figure 3. The Leading Circle Model describes a process involving two closely coupled stimuli which are applied to the center of a cardiac tissue preparation. Owing to intrinsic electrical heterogeneities of the tissue, not all areas will recover in time to be excited by the second stimulus; this creates areas of refractory tissue which essentially act as obstacles for the second propagating impulse. The impulse is forced to circumvent the refractory tissue and travel counterclockwise until it arrives back to the area of refractory tissue which by this time has recovered and can once again be excited by the returning impulse, therefore establishing a re-entrant arrhythmia circuit. The following sections discuss another functional re-entrant arrhythmia mechanism, transmural dispersion of repolarization (TDR), which similarly relies on

Control Preparation

Proarrhythmic Preparation

Single electrical impulse
delivered to the centre of the
tissue preparation

Premature extra
stimulus delivered to the
tissue preparation

Zone of refractory tissue
blocks conduction of
the impulses

Spread of impulse
throughout the tissue
preparation

Electrical wavefront
travels anticlockwise
until arriving at the zone
of refractory tissue, which
by this point has
recovered from excitation
and is able to conduct the
impulse

Electrical wavefront
circumvents zone of
refractory tissue

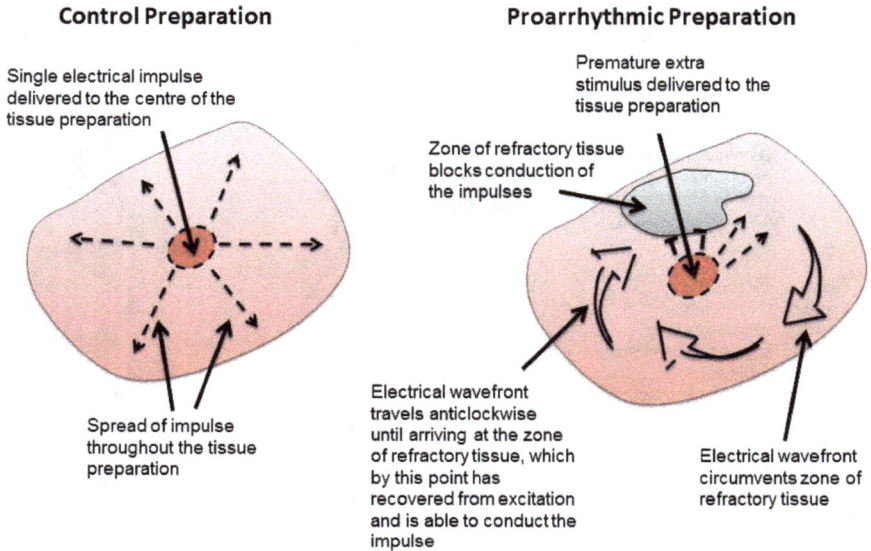

Figure 3:   The Leading Circle Model of arrhythmogenic re-entry.

the heart's electrophysiological heterogeneity to generate arrhythmias. It appears that TDR may play a central role in the generation of ventricular arrhythmias in a variety of different clinical disorders, including drug-induced QT prolongation and proarrhythmia.

Transmural Dispersion of Repolarization

In mammalian hearts, cardiac repolarization follows tightly regulated patterns, from the epicardium to endocardium and from the apex to base — it is now widely agreed that these patterns help to maintain cardiac pump function by providing an important safeguard against arrhythmias. In order to facilitate this orderly pattern of repolarization in the heart, cardiac myocytes express different densities of ion channels, particularly K^+ channels, that result in APs of varying durations throughout the heart. The crucial epicardial to endocardial and apex to base repolarization gradients are governed by differences in AP duration (APD) in the heart; endocardial APD is longer than epicardial APD, and basal APD is longer than apical APD.

As early as the start of the 19th century, a report emerged which described different time courses of repolarization across the surface of the ventricle. In 1913 Mines, a prominent Cambridge physiologist, described that repolarization was longer at the base compared to the apex of the heart. An important study conducted in the mid-1970s was amongst the first to describe a transmural difference in repolarization, in which AP recordings taken from regions in the center of a cardiac muscle preparation had longer APDs than those recorded from either epicardial or endocardial sites. Investigations in larger mammalian hearts, particularly the canine heart, have reported the presence of a third population of cells occurring within the thickness of the ventricular wall, flanked either side by endocardial and epicardial myocytes, mid-myocardial cells (M-cells) (Figure 4) (Antzelevitch *et al.*, 1991).

It is thought that the precise anatomical location of M-cells varies throughout the heart, with studies describing their presence in subendocardial layers of the anterior ventricle and in subepicardial layers of the posterior ventricle. Due to a lack of I_{Ks} and a higher degree

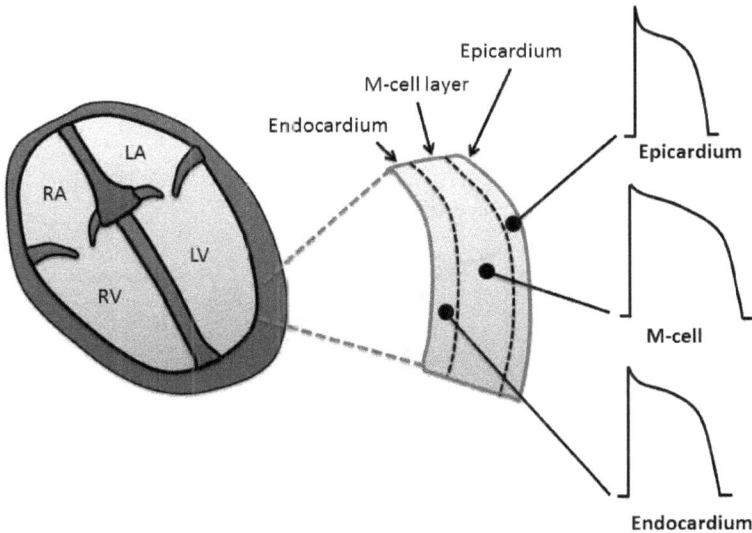

Figure 4: The heterogeneity of ventricular repolarization.

of late Na^+ current $(I_{Na,L})$, M-cells have the longest APDs, and they are exquisitely sensitive to reductions in heart rate and drugs that block the HERG K^+ channel, by exhibiting disproportionately lengthened APDs compared to neighboring endocardial or epicardial cells.

Transmural dispersion of repolarization is measured as the difference between the longest and shortest APDs and experimental conditions that mimic drug-induced QT prolongation lead to an increase in TDR (Figure 5) and the appearance of arrhythmias. Increases in TDR have been implicated in the pathogenesis of Brugada syndrome and congenital LQTS; experimental models that have been created to indirectly model these human cardiac diseases all display an increased TDR, owing primarily to the preferential prolongation of the M-cell APD.

An increase in TDR is thought to increase the susceptibility of the heart to the development of arrhythmias by re-entry mechanisms. An elegant study by Akar and colleagues recorded transmural APs in ventricular tissue preparations (Akar *et al.*, 2002). A surrogate model of drug-induced QT prolongation and proarrhythmia, through the use of

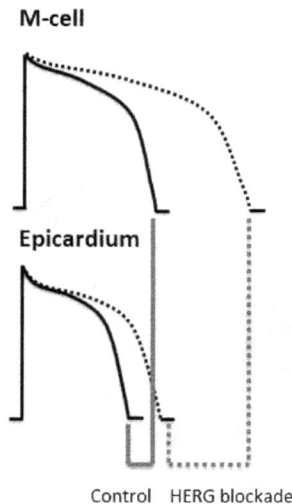

Figure 5:   An illustration of the transmural dispersion of repolarization, measured by the difference between M-cell and epicardial action potential durations, increased due to HERG blockade.

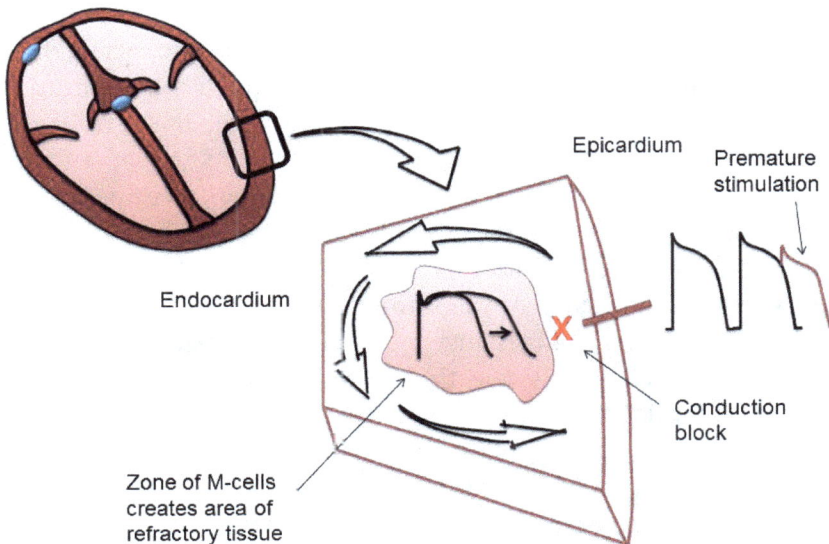

Figure 6: The transmural dispersion model of arrhythmia induction and perpetuation.

sotalol (a Class III antiarrhythmic drug that blocks the HERG K^+ channel) was used to observe patterns of activation and recovery during arrhythmias. The M-cells formed discrete zones of refractory tissue owing to the excessive prolongation of their APDs following sotalol administration. Premature depolarizations applied to the epicardial surface were blocked by the M-cell zones and forced to propagate around these areas of conduction block until they arrived back at their point of origin, by which time the M-cell zones had recovered from excitability and were now able to conduct the impulse, thereby completing the first circuit of arrhythmogenic re-entry (Figure 6).

How does Action Potential and QT Prolongation Generate Arrhythmias?

As discussed in the previous sections, triggering events, such as EADs, and the presence of an appropriate substrate, in the form of an abnormal TDR, both play central roles in the initiation and propagation of cardiac arrhythmias, particularly in the setting of QT prolongation. In the case of congenital LQTS and drug-induced QT prolongation, both factors appear to play a role in the induction of arrhythmias, and they form the basis of the trigger-substrate model of arrhythmia induction. In the trigger-substrate model, reduced repolarization prolongs the cardiac AP and QT interval, which increases the likelihood of EAD and triggered beat generation (the arrhythmia trigger). At the same time, impaired repolarization induces significant changes in ventricular repolarization gradients (the TDR) which predispose the heart to re-entrant arrhythmias (the arrhythmia substrate). According to the trigger-substrate model, ventricular arrhythmias are initiated when a triggered beat occurs in the setting of a significantly altered dispersion of repolarization. The trigger-substrate model of arrhythmia induction is illustrated in Figure 7.

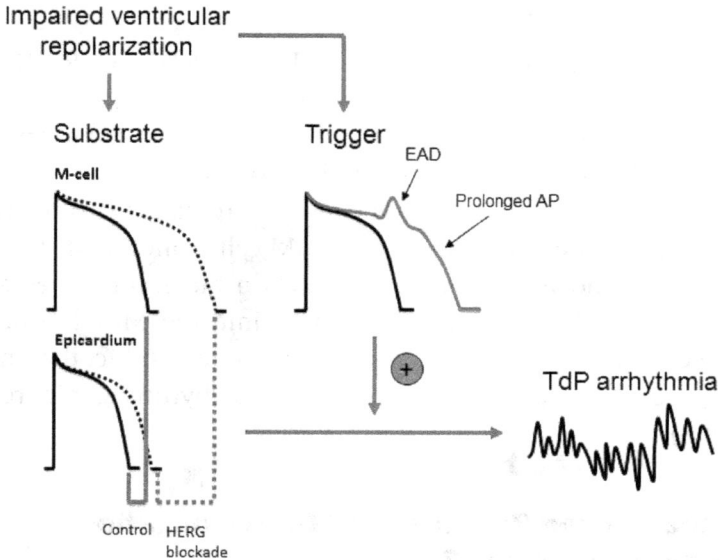

Figure 7: The trigger-substrate model of arrhythmia induction associated with impaired repolarization.

Does the M-Cell Play a Role in Arrhythmia Induction in Humans?

Despite a large number of compelling experimental studies that have demonstrated that M-cells and a TDR appear to help generate arrhythmias, several reports have suggested that the precise role of M-cells in establishing arrhythmias in intact hearts, including the human heart, is unclear (Anyukhovsky *et al.*, 1999; Conrath *et al.*, 2004; Opthof *et al.*, 2007).

The uncertain role of the M-cell in driving cardiac arrhythmias arises from a series of studies that have consistently failed to record M-cells in the intact heart. Although M-cell electrical activity has been recorded from isolated single cells and ventricular tissue preparations, investigations in the intact porcine (Rodriguez-Sinovas *et al.*, 1997), canine (Opthof *et al.*, 2007) and even human heart (Opthof, 2006; Taggart *et al.*, 2003) have failed to report the existence of M-cell-driven repolarization gradients. It has been proposed that cellular electrical (electrotonic) interactions present in intact hearts reduce the reportedly large discrepancies in APDs transmurally within the ventricle (Conrath *et al.*, 2004).

From work dating back to the 1970s in isolated tissue preparations, electrical heterogeneity was identified in Purkinje fibers in which proximal fibers had significantly longer repolarizing times than distal fibers coupled to working myocardium (Myerburg *et al.*, 1970). Since these important findings, the role of cardiac tissue in reducing repolarization times and gradients through electrotonic interactions has been suggested as a possible mechanism underlying the differences in repolarization times reported in a range of experimental preparations. It is worthy to note that as one moves from the single cell to the whole organ level, ventricular repolarization times significantly decrease, implicating a crucial role of electrotonic coupling in reducing repolarization times and heterogeneities. These effects could mask M-cells and help to explain discrepancies in findings between intact heart and isolated tissue and single-cell studies. The greater the degree of uncoupling of cells from neighboring regions could permit them to display repolarization times governed primarily by their ion channel repertoire; in the case of M-cells, a lack of I_{Ks} and an increased $I_{Na,L}$ could contribute to marked increases in APD compared to neighboring epicardial or endocardial regions as seen in isolated tissue preparations.

Another factor that may contribute to the presence of a zone of delayed repolarization in the middle of the ventricular wall is the concept that M-cells are a functionally discrete cell population and that M-cell-driven changes in TDR can only appear under conditions of perturbed repolarization. In this respect, in keeping with findings from intact heart studies, it would be hard to detect M-cells and noticeable repolarization gradients under baseline conditions.

A great deal of the work performed so far into repolarization heterogeneity and its role in arrhythmias and SCD has been conducted in larger mammalian hearts; similarities between canine and human hearts in terms of AP waveforms and ionic currents, for example, make the canine heart an attractive experimental model. However, other models such as the genetically-amenable mouse have been proven to be powerful tools to study the mechanisms underlying arrhythmias when repolarization is impaired. The following sections describe several studies, performed in the mouse heart, that have increased our understanding of how arrhythmias may arise in the setting of QT prolongation.

Using Mouse Models to Study Arrhythmia Mechanisms

The genetically amenable mouse is an attractive model to study the mechanisms underlying arrhythmias; studies have demonstrated that this model system can recapitulate not only arrhythmias, but also accompanying changes in repolarization phenomena such as EADs and alterations in the dispersion of repolarization. In addition to the mouse heart, we have recently witnessed the emergence of two other powerful model systems in which to study human arrhythmias — the transgenic rabbit heart (Brunner *et al.*, 2008) and the genetically amenable zebrafish heart (Milan *et al.*, 2003; 2006).

The mouse model is a major system in which to study the mechanisms underlying cardiac arrhythmias and the direct consequences of ion channel mutations on cardiac physiology; experiments using mouse models have been able to provide a direct link between mutations seen in congenital long QT syndrome patients and cardiac arrhythmias. A number of mouse models have thus far been developed which recapitulate a range of human arrhythmias (Killeen *et al.*, 2008a). A large body of evidence has demonstrated not only the ability of mouse models to generate and maintain a range of arrhythmias but also to display a number of important proarrhythmia features, including repolarization dispersions and EADs. There are, however, important differences in heart rate, heart size and repolarizing currents between mice and other mammalian species and results from studies conducted using the mouse heart need to be transferred to the clinical setting with caution.

The mouse heart is capable of developing established arrhythmogenic features such as EADs (Fabritz *et al.*, 2003a), DADs (Liu *et al.*, 2006) and changes in transmural AP gradients (Thomas *et al.*, 2007c). In common with studies performed in larger mammalian hearts, these features are strongly associated with arrhythmogenesis. Murine hearts can also develop a broad range of cardiac arrhythmias including monomorphic (Thomas *et al.*, 2007c) and polymorphic ventricular tachycardia (VT) (Fabritz *et al.*, 2003b), and even TdP (Kuo *et al.*, 2001); importantly, these arrhythmias share similar features to the corresponding arrhythmias seen in patients. Furthermore, previous studies have shown that genetic mouse models corresponding to congenital LQTS subtypes 3 and 5 (Balasubramaniam *et al.*, 2003; Head *et al.*, 2005), recapitulate features of these human electrical disorders seen in the clinic. Finally, the murine heart exhibits similar responses to pharmacological agents compared to other mammalian hearts including increases in rate in response to isoproterenol (Liu *et al.*, 2006) and arrhythmia suppression with class I (Stokoe *et al.*, 2007) and class IV (Thomas *et al.*, 2007c) antiarrhythmics. With these findings in mind the mouse is a strong model system for further understanding the mechanisms underlying human arrhythmias.

The mouse heart and human heart share many important physiological properties. Structurally, the SA and AV nodes and His-Purkinje system are very similar in mice and in other mammalian systems (Rentschler *et al.*, 2001). Additionally, the AP conduction velocity is identical in murine and canine hearts and AP depolarization and repolarization patterns in mice and other mammalian hearts are similar. The mouse heart also displays APD heterogeneity (Wang *et al.*, 2006). Numerous studies have demonstrated the existence of both transmural and apico-basal repolarization gradients in the mouse heart and arrhythmogenesis in response to alteration of these gradients, similar to findings first identified in larger mammalian hearts. Repolarization times are shorter in epicardial compared to endocardial regions and in apical compared to basal regions (London *et al.*, 2007; Killeen *et al.*, 2007a). In the mouse heart such ventricular APD heterogeneity is largely due to transmural and apico-basal gradients of I_{to} (London *et al.*, 2007; Killeen *et al.*, 2007a; Wang *et al.*, 2006). Finally the mouse and human hearts share nearly identical ionic currents (Nerbonne *et al.*, 2001). Despite these similarities, however, there are some striking differences between mouse and human hearts.

Resting heart rates in the mouse range from 600–700 beats per minute, which is over ten times the human resting heart rate. Action potential waveforms are also different in mice and humans: APs recorded from the mouse heart are significantly shorter than human APs with APDs at 90% (APD_{90}) ranging from 25–42 ms (Killeen *et al.*, 2007a). Action potentials from the mouse heart also lack a well-defined plateau region. Repolarization phases in the human heart are heavily reliant upon the rapid and slow components of the delayed rectifier K^+ channel currents (I_{Kr} and I_{Ks}, respectively), whereas in the adult mouse heart I_{to} is the prominent repolarizing current. As discussed in Chapter 2, the roles that I_{Kr} and I_{Ks} play in cardiac repolarization in the mouse heart are unclear.

Experimental Studies Exploring the Relationship Between Changes in Transmural Repolarization Gradients and Arrhythmias in Mouse Hearts

A number of studies have explored for an association between alterations in transmural repolarization gradients and the incidence of ventricular arrhythmias in genetic mouse models corresponding to congenital LQTS. Repolarization abnormalities and arrhythmias have been reported in a genetically modified Long QT Syndrome type 3 (LQT3) mouse model (Thomas *et al.*, 2007a). LQT3 mice exhibited prolonged epicardial APDs in the presence of unaltered endocardial repolarization times, resulting in a loss of the transmural repolarization gradient that is ordinarily present in the mouse heart (Thomas *et al.*, 2007a).

Programmed electrical stimulation (PES; a common experimental technique that is used to provoke arrhythmias) revealed a high incidence of arrhythmias and, following the induction of AV block, the mice also displayed frequent EADs which were immediately followed by episodes arrhythmias (Thomas *et al.*, 2007a). Treatment with varying concentrations of the non-selective beta-adrenoceptor antagonist, propranolol, produced conditions in which the specific contributions of both EADs and changes in repolarization gradients to arrhythmogenesis could be determined (Thomas *et al.*, 2007b). Low concentrations (100 nM) of propranolol reduced epicardial APD and suppressed EADs alongside spontaneously-occurring and provoked arrhythmias (Thomas *et al.*, 2007b). Higher concentrations (1 µM), despite eliminating EADs and spontaneous arrhythmias, increased the susceptibility of the hearts to provoked arrhythmias. These paradoxical findings could be explained following examination of epicardial and endocardial repolarization times which revealed that 100 nM propranolol corrected the repolarization gradient through selective reduction of epicardial APD while 1 µM propranolol augmented the gradient via prolongation of epicardial yet reduction of endocardial APD (Thomas *et al.*, 2007b). Similar differential actions of propranolol upon ventricular epicardial and endocardial repolarization have also been reported in the canine ventricular wedge preparation (Krishnan and Antzelevitch, 1991) and provide a possible mechanistic explanation to clinical findings in LQT3 patients who appear to derive less antiarrhythmic benefit from beta-adrenoceptor antagonists compared to LQT1 or LQT2 patients.

Following targeted disruption of the KCNE1 gene, a mouse model of LQT5 was established in which hearts displayed impaired epicardial repolarization in addition to EADs, triggered activity, arrythmias and marked reductions in the transmural repolarization gradient (Thomas *et al.*, 2007c). Administration of nifedipine (a selective blocker of the L-type Ca^{2+} channel) produced a cascade of antiarrhythmic effects by correcting deficits in epicardial repolarization, restoring the physiological repolarization gradient, and eliminating EADs and triggered activity (Thomas *et al.*, 2007c).

In addition to the above research in genetically modified mouse hearts, modeling various forms of congenital LQTS, our understanding of arrhythmia mechanisms has increased from studies that have examined the effects of hypokalemia on the mouse heart. Hypokalemia is an important, acquired cause of arrhythmias in the setting of QT prolongation. Experiments studying hypokalemia's proarrhythmic effects on the heart have reinforced many key principles of arrhythmogenesis and they thus serve as important case studies for further understanding how arrhythmias may arise and how they may be prevented.

Arrhythmia Mechanisms and Novel Antiarrhythmic Approaches Identified Using the Hypokalemic Mouse Model

Hypokalemia is an important risk factor for the induction of drug-induced arrhythmias; a drug's effects on prolonging the QT interval and inducing arrhythmias may be significantly amplified in the setting of hypokalemia. At the clinical level, hypokalemia has been shown to cause QT prolongation and at the cellular level it has been shown to reduce repolarizing K^+ channel currents (Yang and Roden, 1996; Yang *et al.*, 1997). However, despite these clinical and experimental observations, the precise mechanisms underlying the proarrhythmic effects of hypokalemia were, until recently, unknown. In the following sections a series of studies which specifically assessed the effects of hypokalemia on the heart and identified several antiarrhythmic approaches are described. These discussions are important not only due to the central role that hypokalemia plays in drug-induced QT prolongation, but also because they serve as powerful case studies for further understanding the mechanisms of ventricular arrhythmias.

In isolated hearts subjected to artificial pacing, AP recordings from the ventricular epicardial and endocardial surface demonstrated a baseline, physiological transmural repolarization gradient of approximately 14 ms (Killeen *et al.*, 2007b). Progressive reductions in $[K^+]_o$ to induce hypokalemia in isolated hearts evoked notable prolongation of ventricular repolarization times; epicardial APD recorded at baseline (with a physiological $[K^+]_o$ of 5.2 mM) increased from 37.2 ms to 58.4 ms and 67.7 ms following perfusion of hearts with solutions containing 4 mM and 3 mM $[K^+]_o$, respectively. Moreover, preferential prolongation of the epicardial APD was seen in the presence of hypokalemic solutions; although both the epicardial and endocardial APD significantly increased in the setting of hypokalemia, epicardial APD_{90} increased by 29.5 ms whereas endocardial APD_{90} increased by only 11.3 ms with 3 mM $[K^+]_o$. These prominent effects reduced, and reversed, the physiological repolarization gradient from 14 to −3.4 ms (Killeen *et al.*, 2007b).

To shed light on these effects of hypokalemic solutions on ventricular repolarization in the mouse heart, a series of cellular experiments were conducted in epicardial and endocardial myocytes to assess for potential changes in repolarizing K^+ channel currents in the setting of hypokalemia (Killeen *et al.*, 2007b). Baseline recordings revealed a significantly greater degree of I_{to} in epidcardial compared to endocardial cells, which undoubtedly contributed to the shorter repolarization times recorded from epicardial versus endocardial surfaces of the isolated hearts. When $[K^+]_o$ was reduced to mimic clinical hypokalemia, epicardial I_{to} was significantly reduced but no such changes were seen in endocardial cells (Killeen *et al.*, 2007a). These findings correlate to the preferential lengthening of epicardial APD seen in isolated hearts and strongly implicate I_{to} as an important mediator of hypokalemia's proarrhythmic effects.

Further experiments were conducted in spontaneously beating hearts to provoke the generation of arrhythmogenic phenomena. Isolated hearts that are not subjected to artificial pacing typically exhibit reduced heart rates compared to those seen *in vivo*; in the mouse heart, for example, the cycle length of spontaneously beating preparations is approximately 334 ms (corresponding to a heart rate of 170 beats per minute [bpm]) compared to a basic cycle length of 125 ms (480 bpm) that is used to mimic the physiological, *in vivo* heart rate of the mouse. The use of spontaneously beating hearts has been exploited as an effective means of increasing a heart's susceptibility to arrhythmias. Perfusing hearts with hypokalemic solutions led to the appearance of EADs (at 4 mM $[K^+]_o$) in addition to triggered beats and episodes of non-sustained and sustained VT (at 3 mM $[K^+]_o$) (Killeen *et al.*, 2007b) (Figure 8). Figure 9 illustrates an example of a spontaneously-occurring arrhythmia in a hypokalemic heart in which a short-long-short sequence, a pattern commonly seen in human cases of TdP, is seen immediately prior to the arrhythmic. Over recording times exceeding five hours, EADs were seen in 62.1% of all APs recorded whilst arrhythmias were seen in 19.1% of APs (Killeen *et al.*, 2007a). These findings of spontaneous arrhythmias in the setting of hypokalemia were corroborated through the use of PES in which arrhythmias were readily induced in 28% of hearts at 4 mM $[K^+]_o$. Of note, this 28% incidence of arrhythmias with a 4 mM hypokalemic solution (representing a 1 mM reduction in $[K^+]_o$) correlates strongly with findings from a large clinical study. The Multiple Risk Factor Intervention Trial demonstrated a remarkably similar incidence of ventricular arrhythmias amongst male hypertensive patients administered diuretics — a 28% increase in ventricular arrhythmias was seen with every 1 mM reduction in serum K^+ levels (Cohen *et al.*, 1987). When $[K^+]_o$ was reduced to 3 mM, the incidence of PES-induced ventricular arrhythmias was much higher

Control Preparation: Normokalemia (5.2 mM [K$^+$]$_o$)

Proarrhythmic Preparation: Hypokalemia (3 mM [K$^+$]$_o$)

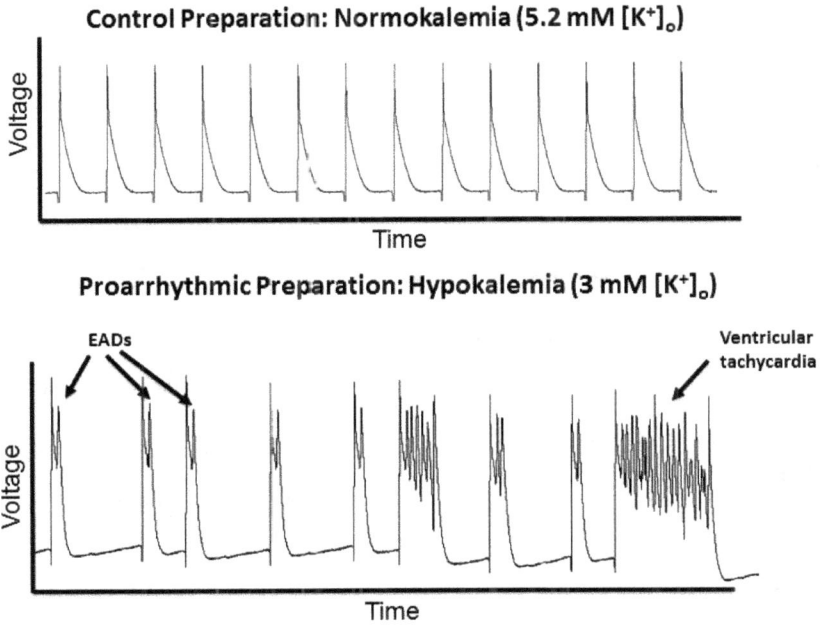

Figure 8: Experimental recordings of early after depolarizations and arrhythmias in the setting of hypokalemia.

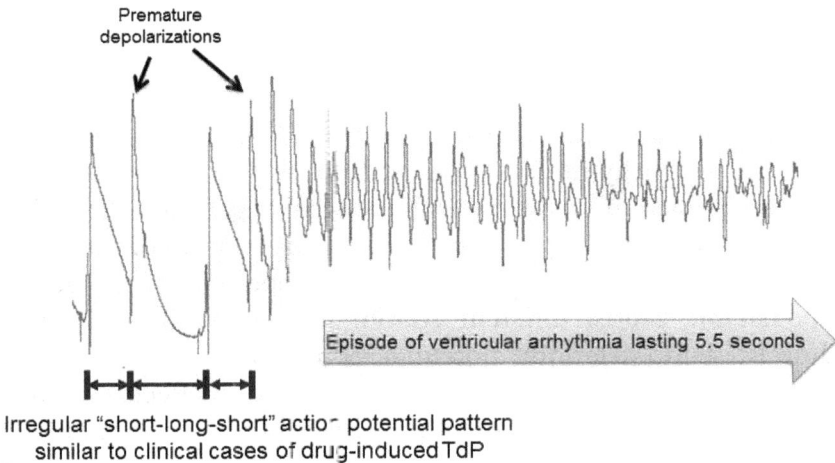

Irregular "short-long-short" action potential pattern similar to clinical cases of drug-induced TdP

Figure 9: A spontaneously occurring arrhythmia recorded from a hypokalemic cardiac preparation.

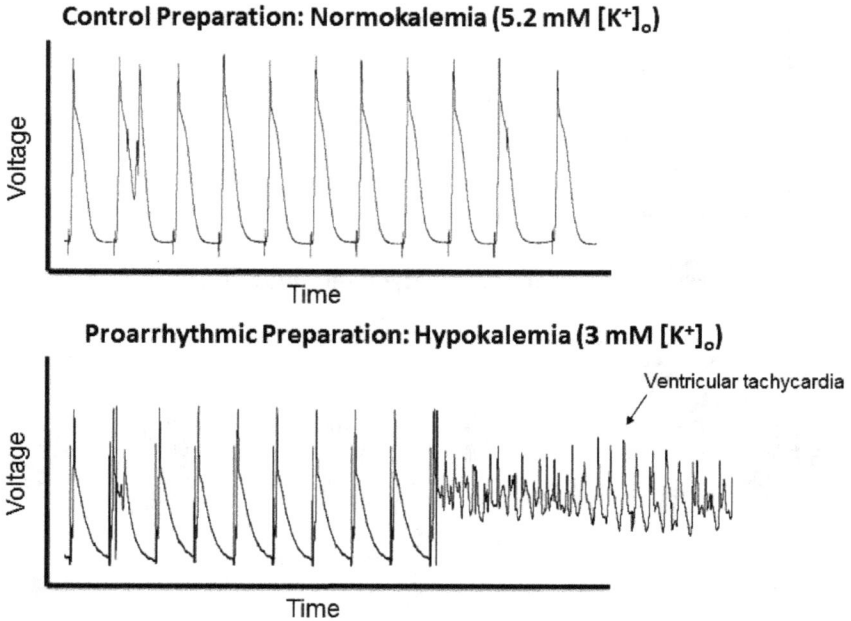

Control Preparation: Normokalemia (5.2 mM [K⁺]ₒ)

Proarrhythmic Preparation: Hypokalemia (3 mM [K⁺]ₒ)

Figure 10:   Provoked ventricular arrhythmias in a hypokalemic preparation.

(arrhythmias were recorded from 81% of hearts) (Killeen *et al.*, 2007b) (Figure 10).

Calcium channels are considered to play an important role in the initiation of arrhythmias through generating EADs; nifedipine was therefore administered to hypokalemic hearts to explore for its potential antiarrhythmic effects and to further understand the precise interaction between EAD-induced triggered activity and altered dispersions of repolarization in the generation of ventricular arrhythmias (Killeen *et al.*, 2007a). In spontaneously beating hypokalemic hearts, different concentrations of nifedipine were administered to determine potential reductions in the incidence of EADs. While a low concentration (10 nM) had no effect, a medium concentration (100 nM) of nifedipine halved the incidence of EADs to 28.3% and reduced the rate of arrhythmias to 1.2%; an even higher nifedipine concentration (1 µM) completely abolished EADs and arrhythmias (Killeen *et al.*, 2007a). In experiments using PES to

Hypokalemia [3 mM [K⁺]ₒ) + nifedipine (1 μM)

Hypokalemia (3 mM [K⁺]ₒ) + nicorandil (20 μM)

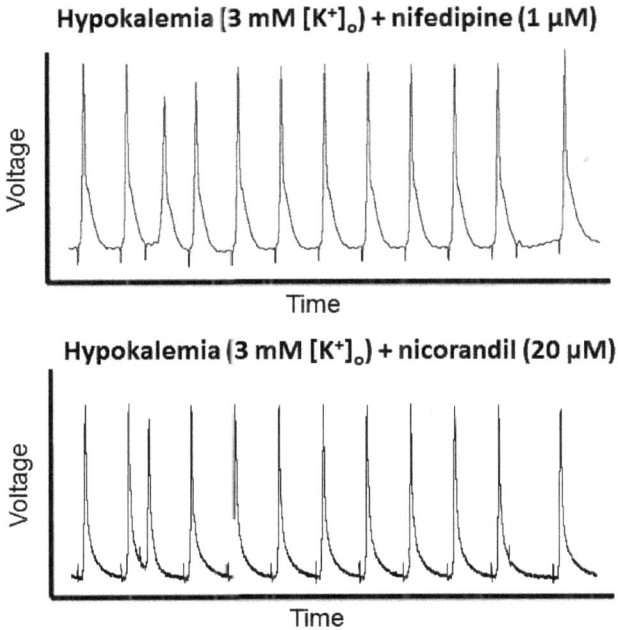

Figure 11: The antiarrhythmic effects of different pharmacological agents in hypokalemic preparations.

provoke arrhythmias, slightly different antiarrhythmic findings were observed: whereas 10 nM nifedipine similarly failed to prevent arrhythmias, administration of 100 nM nifedipine also did not exert any antiarrhythmic effects in contrast to its ability to reduce EADs and arrhythmias in spontaneously beating hearts. However, PES failed to induce arrhythmias in hearts given the highest nifedipine concentration (1 μM) (Figure 11).

The effects of nifedipine on the epidcardial and endocardial APD were measured to determine if antiarrhythmic effects could be explained by changes in the transmural repolarization gradient. Low and medium nifedipine concentrations did not have any effect on APDs and thus the abnormal repolarization gradient, seen with hypokalemia, remained the same. However, the highest nifedipine concentration selectively, and significantly, reduced the epicardial APD from 66.1 to 46.2 ms (no changes in endocardial APD were seen); this effect led to a dramatic change, and restoration, of the repolarization gradient from −5.9 to 15.5 ms (Killeen *et al.*, 2007a).

Similar findings were also seen with an inhibitor of calmodulin kinase (CaMK) type II, KN-93. A number of different studies have identified CaMKII as a novel proarrhythmic signaling molecule in a range of clinical disorders including congenital LQTS, cardiac hypertrophy, and cardiomyopathy. Initially activated by raised levels of intracellular Ca^{2+}, CaMKII appears to be an important regulator of the L-type Ca^{2+} channel; in a genetically modified mouse model of cardiac hypertrophy, generated through raised CaMKII activity, L-type Ca^{2+} channels had an increased probability of opening (Wu *et al.*, 2002) which could lead to a higher rate of EADs and arrhythmias. Additionally in an arrhythmogenic rabbit heart model that showed increased CaMKII activity, pharmacological inhibition of CaMKII exerted antiarrhythmic effects (Anderson *et al.*, 1998). In hypokalemic mouse hearts KN-93 suppressed EADs, triggered activity, and arrhythmias but the drug failed to exert similar antiarrhythmic effects in preparations provoked using PES. Analysis of KN-93's effects on the APD revealed that it did not cause any significant changes in either epicardial or endocardial APD and it therefore preserved the abnormal repolarization gradient seen in the setting of hypokalemia.

These findings with nifedipine and KN-93 have important implications for our understanding of how drug-induced arrhythmias arise and in identifying potential antiarrhythmic therapeutic strategies. As we saw with the low and medium concentrations of nifedipine, while they significantly reduced arrhythmias, most likely through a reduction in EADs, these concentrations did not prevent provoked arrhythmias using PES. Also, the low and medium nifedipine concentrations did not have any effect on the abnormal repolarization gradient seen in hypokalemic hearts, while the highest concentration completely restored the gradient to a normal value. This study therefore implicates both EADs and abnormal repolarization gradients in the generation of arrhythmias in which the presence of both is necessary for acquired ventricular arrhythmias seen with hypokalemia. While suppression of EADs alone (i.e. the trigger) can prevent arrhythmias, if the underlying arrhythmogenic repolarization gradient remains present (i.e. substrate), arrhythmias may still occur if an artificial premature stimulus is applied. As seen with the highest concentration of nifedipine, only through suppression of EADs and the restoration of the repolarization gradient can strong antiarrhythmic effects be observed.

An alternative pharmacological approach to suppress ventricular arrhythmias in the setting of delayed repolarization due to acquired conditions (e.g. drug therapy or hypokalemia) is the activation of repolarizing K^+ channel currents. Drugs that are capable of activating, and hence increasing, repolarization K^+ channel currents are an attractive antiarrhythmic approach as they would be expected to increase the level of repolarization and counter APD and QT prolongation. As discussed in the sections above, delayed repolarization is an important mediator of ventricular arrhythmias through the facilitation of EAD induction and the alteration of repolarizing gradients.

The hypokalemic mouse model was used to assess the antiarrhythmic effects of two different K^+ channel activators, nicorandil and NS1643. Nicorandil is an activator of the K_{ATP} K^+ channel and it has been extensively used for the management of angina. In addition to these therapeutic effects, a series of studies have also described its antiarrhythmic effects in the setting of congenital LQTS (Shimizu and Antzelevitch, 2000; Shimizu et al., 1998). Nicorandil therefore has the potential to be an effective antiarrhythmic drug in the setting of other causes of QT prolongation and impaired repolarization. NS1643 is an experimental drug that has been shown to activate the HERG K^+ channel and reduce the APD in isolated cells (Hansen et al., 2006). Studies using these drugs in the mouse model not only further demonstrate the causal relationship between delayed repolarization and arrhythmias, but also identify two promising novel antiarrhythmic approaches.

Both nicorandil and NS1643 exerted notable antiarrhythmic effects in spontaneously beating hypokalemic hearts. NS1643 abolished EADs, triggered activity, and ventricular arrhythmias in 54% of preparations whilst nicorandil suppressed arrhythmias in 83% of hearts (Figure 11) (Killeen *et al.*, 2008b). The antiarrhythmic efficacies of nicorandil and NS1643 were correlated to their effects on repolarization times. Nicorandil evoked a significant reduction in epicardial repolarization times, thereby restoring the transmural repolarization gradient. Although NS1643 had similar effects on ventricular repolarization, it was not as effective as nicorandil at reducing prolonged APDs and correcting the repolarization gradient in the setting of hypokalemia. These findings demonstrated for the first time the antiarrhythmic efficacy of K$^+$ channel activation in the setting of hypokalemia. NS1643 and nicorandil exerted antiarrhythmic actions through the suppression of EADs, reductions in APD, and the restoration of the repolarization gradient.

The outcomes of experimental studies that assess the antiarrhythmic effects of K$^+$ channel activators are greatly influenced by the model system used. In the study of nicorandil and NS1643 in hypokalemic mouse hearts, nicorandil was more effective than NS1643 in suppressing arrhythmias. These effects are likely to result from different levels of I_{KATP} and I_{Kr} in the mouse heart and the contribution of these two ion channels to cardiac repolarization in the mouse. These differences in cardiac electrophysiology between species are important factors that should be considered when assessing the pharmacological effects of drugs on the heart.

Changes in repolarization gradients, in large as well as small hearts, constitute an important proarrhythmic mechanism of action, facilitating functional re-entry and perpetuating arrhythmias. Issues remain to be resolved when measuring TDR in the canine and other larger hearts, although the evidence to date points to differences in experimental techniques and conditions in contributing to discrepancies in findings between cellular, tissue and intact heart preparations. Additionally, despite the small size of the mouse heart, it is capable of displaying important proarrhythmic mechanisms seen in much larger hearts, including changes in transmural repolarization gradients and triggering factors such as EADs and DADs; the mouse heart has therefore emerged as a powerful tool for studying arrhythmia mechanisms. Differences in heart rates and repolarizing currents between mice and humans, however, merit caution when transferring findings from mouse studies to the clinic.

Summary

The mechanisms underlying cardiac arrhythmias in the setting of QT prolongation are complex. The mammalian heart is electrically heterogenous and APs recorded from different locations have distinct morphologies and durations. Differences in APD between neighboring regions in the heart create repolarization gradients which ordinarily provide an important defence against arrhythmias. A large body of evidence from a series of experimental studies indicates that disrupting these physiological repolarization gradients greatly increases the heart's susceptibility to arrhythmias by generating a proarrhythmic substrate. Triggered activity, due to afterdepolarizations, occurring in the presence of an appropriate substrate is the basis of the trigger–substrate model of arrhythmia induction which is considered to be one of the main mechanisms contributing to arrhythmias that occur in patients with a prolonged QT interval.

References

Akar, F. *et al.* (2002). Unique topographical distribution of M cells underlies re-entrant mechanism of torsade de pointes in the long-QT syndrome. *Circulation*, **105**, 1247–1253.

Anderson, M. *et al.* (1998). KN-93, an inhibitor of multifunctional Ca^{++}/calmodulin-dependent protein kinase, decreases early afterdepolarizationsin the rabbit heart. *J Pharmacol Exp Ther*, **287**, 996–1006.

Antzelevitch, C. *et al.* (1991). Heterogeneity within the ventricular wall. Electrophysiology and pharmacology of epicardial, endocardial, and M cells. *Circ Res*, **69**, 1427–1449.

Anyukhovsky, E. *et al.* (1999). The controversial M cell. *J Cardiovasc Electrophysiol*, **10**, 244–260.

Balasubramaniam, R. *et al.* (2003). Electrogram prolongation and nifedipine-suppressible ventricular arrhythmias in mice following targeted disruption of KCNE1. *J Physiol*, **552**, 535–546.

Benson, D. *et al.* (2003). Congenital sick sinus syndrome caused by recessive mutations in the cardiac sodium channel gene (SCN5A). *J Clin Invest,* **112,** 1019–1028.

Brunner, M. *et al.* (2008). Mechanisms of cardiac arrhythmias and sudden death in transgenic rabbits with long QT syndrome. *J Clin Invest,* **118,** 2246–2259.

Cohen, J. *et al.* (1987). Diuretics, serum potassium and ventricular arrhythmias in the Multiple Risk Factor Intervention Trial. *Am J Cardiol,* **60,** 548–554.

Conrath, C. *et al.* (2004). Intercellular coupling through gap junctions masks M cells in the human heart. *Cardiovasc Res,* **62,** 407–414.

Fabritz, L. *et al.* (2003a). Prolonged action potential durations, increased dispersion of repolarization, and polymorphic ventricular tachycardia in a mouse model of proarrhythmia. *Basic Res Cardiol,* **98,** 25–32.

Fabritz, L. *et al.* (2003b). Effect of pacing and mexiletine on dispersion of repolarisation and arrhythmias in Delta KPQ SCN5A (long QT3) mice. *Cardiovasc Res,* **57,** 1085–1093.

Hansen, R. *et al.* (2006). Activation of human ether-a-go-go-related gene potassium channels by the diphenylurea 1,3-bis-(2-hydroxy-5-trifluoromethyl-phenyl)-urea (NS1643). *Mol Pharmacol,* **69,** 266–277.

Head, C. *et al.* (2005). Paced electrogram fractionation analysis of arrhythmogenic tendency in KPQ Scn5a mice. *J Cardiovasc Electrophysiol,* **16,** 1329–1340.

Kannel, W. *et al.* (1987). Sudden death risk in overt coronary heart disease: the Framingham Study. *Am Heart J,* **113,** 799–804.

Killeen, M. *et al.* (2007a). Separation of early afterdepolarizations from arrhythmogenic substrate in the isolated perfused hypokalaemic murine heart through modifiers of calcium homeostasis. *Acta Physiol (Oxf),* **191,** 43–58.

Killeen, M. *et al.* (2007b). Arrhythmogenic mechanisms in the isolated perfused hypokalaemic murine heart. *Acta Physiol (Oxf),* **189,** 33–46.

Killeen, M. *et al.* (2008a). Mouse models of human arrhythmia syndromes. *Acta Physiol (Oxf),* **192,** 455–469.

Killeen, M. *et al.* (2008b). Effects of potassium channel openers in the isolated perfused murine heart. *Acta Physiol (Oxf),* **193,** 25–36.

Krishnan, S.C. and Antzelevitch, C. (1991). Sodium channel block produces opposite electrophysiological effects in canine ventricular epicardium and endocardium. *Circ Res.* **69**, 277–291.

Kuo, H. *et al.* (2001). A defect in the Kv channel-interacting protein 2 (KChIP2) gene leads to a complete loss of I(to) and confers susceptibility to ventricular tachycardia. *Cell*, **107**, 801–813.

Liu, N. *et al.* (2006). Arrhythmogenesis in catecholaminergic polymorphic ventricular tachycardia: insights from a RyR2 R4496C knock-in mouse model. *Circ Res*, **99**, 292–298.

London, B. *et al.* (2007). Dispersion of repolarization and refractoriness are determinants of arrhythmia phenotype in transgenic mice with long QT. *J Physiol*, **578**, 115–129.

Milan, D. *et al.* (2006). *In vivo* recording of adult zebrafish electrocardiogram and assessment of drug-induced QT prolongation. *Am J Physiol Heart Circ Physiol*, **291**, H259–273.

Milan, D. *et al.* (2003). Drugs that induce repolarization abnormalities cause bradycardia in zebrafish. *Circulation*, **107**, 1355–1358.

Mines, G.R. (1913). On dynamic equilibrium in the heart. *J Physiol*, **46**, 349–383.

Mohler, P. *et al.* (2003) Ankyrin-B mutation causes type 4 long-QT cardiac arrhythmia and sudden cardiac death. *Nature*, **421**, 634–639.

Myerburg, R. *et al.* (1970). On-line measurement of duration of cardiac action potentials and refractory periods. *J Appl Physiol*, **28**, 92–93.

Nerbonne, J. *et al.* (2001). Genetic manipulation of cardiac K(+) channel function in mice: what have we learned, and where do we go from here? *Circ Res*, **89**, 944–956.

NICE. (2000). Guidance on the use of implantable cardioverter defibrillators for arrhythmias. Department of Health, pp.1–15.

Opthof, T. (2006). *In vivo* dispersion in repolarization and arrhythmias in the human heart. *Am J Physiol Heart Circ Physiol*, **290**, 77–78.

Opthof, T. *et al.* (2007). Dispersion of repolarization in canine ventricle and the electrocardiographic T wave: Tp-e interval does not reflect transmural dispersion. *Heart Rhythm*, **4**, 341–348.

Rentschler, S. *et al.* (2001). Visualization and functional characterization of the developing murine cardiac conduction system. *Development*, **128**, 1785–1792.

Roden, D.M. and Hoffman, B.F. (1985). Action potential prolongation and induction of abnormal automaticity by low quinidine concentrations in canine Purkinje fibers. Relationship to potassium and cycle length. *Circ Res*, **56**, 857–867.

Rodriguez-Sinovas, A. *et al.* (1997). Lack of evidence of M-cells in porcine left ventricular myocardium. *Cardiovasc Res*, **33**, 307–313.

Shimizu, W. and Antzelevitch, C. (2000). Effects of a K(+) channel opener to reduce transmural dispersion of repolarization and prevent torsade de pointes in LQT1, LQT2, and LQT3 models of the long-QT syndrome. *Circulation*, **102**, 706–712.

Shimizu, W. *et al.* (1998). Improvement of repolarization abnormalities by a K+ channel opener in the LQT1 form of congenital long-QT syndrome. *Circulation*, **97**, 1581–1588.

Stokoe, K. *et al.* (2007). Effects of flecainide and quinidine on arrhythmogenic properties of Scn5a+/{Delta} murine hearts modelling long QT syndrome 3. *J Physiol*, **578**, 69–84.

Taggart, P. *et al.* (2003). Electrotonic cancellation of transmural electrical gradients in the left ventricle in man. *Prog Biophys Mol Biol*, **82**, 243–254.

Thomas, G. *et al.* (2007a). Effects of L-type Ca^{2+} channel antagonism on ventricular arrhythmogenesis in murine hearts containing a modification in the Scn5a gene modelling human long QT syndrome 3. *J Physiol*, **578**, 85–97.

Thomas, G. *et al.* (2007b). Pharmacological separation of early afterdepolarizations from arrhythmogenic substrate in DeltaKPQ Scn5a murine hearts modelling human long QT 3 syndrome. *Acta Physiol (Oxf)*, **92**, 505–517.

Thomas, G. *et al.* (2007c). Mechanisms of ventricular arrhythmogenesis in mice following targeted disruption of KCNE1 modelling long QT syndrome 5. *J Physiol*, **578**, 99–114.

Wang, Y. *et al.* (2006). Remodeling of early-phase repolarization: a mechanism of abnormal impulse conduction in heart failure. *Circulation*, **113**, 1849–1856.

Willich, S. *et al.* (1987). Circadian variation in the incidence of sudden cardiac death in the Framingham Heart Study population. *Am J Cardiol*, **60**, 801–806.

Wu, Y. *et al.* (2002). Calmoculin kinase II and arrhythmias in a mouse model of cardiac hypertrophy. *Circulation*, **106**, 1288–1293.

Yang, T. and Roden, D.M. (1996) Extracellular potassium modulation of drug block of IKr. Implications for torsade de pointes and reverse use-dependence. *Circulation*, **93**, 407–411.

Yang, T. *et al.* (1997) Rapid inactivation determines the rectification and [K+]o dependence of the rapid component of the delayed rectifier K+ current in cardiac cells. *Circ Res*, **80**, 782–789.

CHAPTER 5

The Mechanisms Underlying Drug-Induced Arrhythmias

Introduction

Experimental models that mimic human arrhythmia syndromes have had a profound impact on our understanding of how arrhythmias arise. A wealth of research has proposed a number of different mechanisms whereby drugs may induce potentially fatal arrhythmias; these studies have shown that many arrhythmia disorders share common mechanisms, such as delays in repolarization, triggered activity, and alterations in repolarization gradients. Building on these principal concepts of arrhythmogenesis, the purpose of this chapter is to more closely examine some of the major mechanisms that are widely considered to underlie drug-induced QT prolongation and proarrhythmia. Although one cellular mechanism appears to play a leading role in this adverse event, vastly different, but equally effective, mechanisms have been reported with a range of drugs.

The Classical Model of Drug-Induced QT Prolongation and Proarrhythmia: HERG Blockade

Pharmacological blockade of the HERG K^+ channel has been acknowledged as one of the prevailing mechanisms underlying drug-induced QT prolongation and proarrhythmia; one study estimated that HERG K$^+$ channel inhibition accounts for over 95% of cases of drug-induced QT prolongation (Lacerda *et al.*, 2008). Accordingly, one of the main aims of a preclinical cardiac safety study is to examine the effects of drugs on this repolarizing K$^+$ channel. Several unique features of the HERG K$^+$ channel are thought to underlie its sensitivity to blockade by a variety of cardiovascular and non-cardiovascular drugs. Ordinarily, K$^+$ channels have a structural attribute, known as the PXP motif, which reduces the size of the ion channel's inner cavity and prevents drugs from becoming trapped within the channel; the HERG K$^+$ channel lacks this structural feature which therefore results in a much larger cavity within the ion channel that can accommodate drugs. Additionally, within the pore region of the HERG K$^+$ channel, two structural features are considered to interact with drugs and to facilitate their binding to the ion channel; in experiments, mutations of these two areas in the HERG K$^+$ channel's pore significantly reduce the ability of drugs to bind to, and block, the ion channel (Tamargo *et al.*, 2004).

When drugs block the HERG K$^+$ channel they significantly reduce the repolarizing capacity of the ventricles and cause prominent AP and QT prolongation. As discussed in Chapter 4, AP prolongation can significantly disrupt cardiac repolarization gradients and generate a proarrhythmic substrate. Drug-induced AP prolongation also leads to the generation of early after depolarizations (EADs) and triggered activity which, if they occur in the setting of an arrhythmia substrate, may result in arrhythmia induction.

Additional Mechanisms Contributing to Drug-Induced Arrhythmias

Despite the fact that direct blockade of the HERG channel appears to underlie the vast majority of cases of drug-induced QT prolongation, from a theoretical standpoint a great many more mechanisms could also delay cardiac repolarization and/or provoke arrhythmias. Indeed, based on our knowledge of congenital Long QT Syndrome (LQTS), in which a range of different mutations affecting multiple cardiac ion channels have been identified, it remains distinctly possible that drug-induced QT prolongation may also arise due to similarly broad mechanisms. Long QT Syndrome type 3 (LQT3), for example, arises from gain-of-function mutations in the cardiac Na^+ channel which lead to a persistent, depolarizing Na^+ current and subsequent delays in ventricular repolarization. As discussed in the sections below, a number of different mechanisms have been demonstrated to underlie drug-induced QT prolongation and proarrhythmia.

Drug-Induction Activation of Depolarizing Ion Channels

Alfuzosin is a small molecule inhibitor of the alpha-1 adrenoceptor that has been approved for the treatment of benign prostatic hyperplasia. The case of alfuzosin-induced cardiac toxicity is an intriguing example of where QT prolongation was not detected in preclinical studies; the safety signal was only detected in a subsequent clinical trial called a Thorough QT (TQT) Study (please see Chapter 6 for a further discussion of the TQT Study). The case of alfuzosin therefore serves as an important example of discordance seen between preclinical and clinical safety studies that may arise during drug development. Preclinical data submitted to the FDA for review consisted of negative findings from a HERG K^+ channel screen, in which the IC_{50} for alfuzosin against HERG was found to be 83 μM and AP prolongation at 1 μM was not seen in Purkinje fiber experiments (Lacerda *et al.*, 2008). Nevertheless, due to the inability to firmly discount a risk of QT prolongation and proarrhythmia with alfuzosin, the FDA required that a TQT study of the drug be conducted; this study tested the effects of 10 mg and 40 mg alfuzosin in healthy volunteers and compared the drug's effects to those seen in subjects administered a positive control drug. The results of the clinical study demonstrated that alfuzosin induced QT prolongation of 7.7 ms. in contrast to the preclinical studies, which represents a positive QT safety signal. To identify the root cause of this discordance, several preclinical experiments were conducted (Lacerda *et al.*, 2008). In part, these experiments confirmed the earlier preclinical results of alfuzosin — very high concentrations of the drug were required to reduce the HERG K^+ channel current. Also, alfuzosin had no effects on the cardiac L-type Ca^{2+} channel current or the transient outward K^+ channel current. However, statistically significant APD prolongation was seen with alfuzosin in a rabbit Purkinje fiber model; reverse-use dependence was observed, in which slower heart rates resulted in a greater degree of APD prolongation (Lacerda *et al.*, 2008). These effects were replicated in isolated heart experiments, in which the AV node was ablated to induce bradycardia, which subsequently demonstrated the ability of alfuzosin to induce QT prolongation. Importantly, alfuzosin induced APD and QT prolongation at a much lower concentration used to block the HERG K^+ channel, which suggested that the drug was unlikely to mediate its effects on repolarization through HERG blockade. Subsequent studies revealed that alfuzosin activated depolarizing Na^+ channels (Lacerda *et al.*, 2008); this effect would be expected to counteract the repolarizing effects of the heart's K^+ channels and lead to a longer time taken for cardiac cells to return to a fully repolarized, resting state.

Ibutilide, a class III antiarrhythmic drug that is known to block the HERG channel, has also been shown to activate a depolarizing ionic current; in keeping with alfuzosin's effects on the Na^+ current, this action of ibutilide may also play a role in its well-recognized ability to induce QT prolongation (Naccarelli *et al.*, 1996). Using isolated human atrial cells, investigators have shown that low concentrations of ibutilide result in an increased inward, depolarizing current (Lee *et al.*, 1998). Although the precise identity of the ion channel that appears to be activated by ibutilide was not revealed, the study's authors proposed that administration of ibutilide resulted in an inward Na^+ current through L-type Ca^{2+} channels (Lee *et al.*, 1998).

Collectively, these findings with alfuzosin and ibutilide highlight an additional mechanism of action that could underlie QT prolongation and lead to a risk of proarrhythmia. Furthermore, these studies emphasize the need to carefully evaluate a drug's effects against a broad range of cardiac ion channels during preclinical cardiac safety screening. As illustrated with alfuzosin, and findings that have emerged from research into congenital LQTS, acute effects on cardiac repolarization may be achieved through a number of different modes of action.

Drug-Induced Changes in Ion Channel Expression

A number of different reports have now demonstrated that a drug's deleterious effects on the HERG K^+ channel may involve both acute and long term mechanisms. A good example of these dual toxic effects against the HERG K^+ channel, which may cause QT prolongation, is the case of fluoxetine, a medication approved for the management of depressive and other psychological disorders, and its metabolite norfluoxetine. Rajamani and colleagues (2006) demonstrated that both fluoxetine and norfluoxetine impair cardiac repolarization not only through direct blockade of the HERG K^+ channel, but also through a novel mode of action in which the drugs reduce the levels of these ionic currents in the cell membrane. Exposure of mammalian cells overexpressing the HERG K^+ channel to fluoxetine and norfluoxentine for 24 hours led to a notable reduction in the levels of these ion channels in cell membranes (Rajamani *et al.*, 2006). Reduced expression of the HERG K^+ channel would be expected to result in a diminished repolarization capacity of myocytes, similar to effects seen with acute blockade of the HERG K^+ channel. Therefore, in the case of fluoxetine and norfluoxetine, their ability to induce QT prolongation appears to be mediated through two different modes of action which both reduce the HERG channel's repolarizing K^+ current. Similar direct and indirect effects on the HERG K^+ channel have also been reported for arsenic trioxide (Ficker *et al.*, 2004). It also appears that these effects on the expression of the HERG K^+ channel are not shared amongst all drugs that directly block the channel; dofetilide and cisapride, for example, are direct inhibitors of HERG but they do not cause a reduction in the levels of the ion channel in cell membranes (Rajamani *et al.*, 2006). Conversely, drugs may reduce the expression of repolarizing K^+ channels without having any direct inhibitory actions on channels themselves.

Pentamidine, a drug used for the treatment of a number of parasitic diseases, has been associated with QT prolongation and several cases of drug-induced torsade de pointes (TdP). In one study of 18 patients, for example, five patients developed a QT interval exceeding 480 ms and TdP was documented in two of these patients (Eisenhauer *et al.*, 1994). Although pentamidine does directly block the HERG K$^+$ channel, its IC$_{50}$ for the channel is over 250 μM — a concentration considerably higher than therapeutic plasma concentrations of the drug. However, long term incubation of cells with pentamidine significantly reduced the levels of HERG K$^+$ channels in cell membranes — repolarizing currents were reduced by up to 85% (Cordes *et al.*, 2005). Therefore, with these findings in mind, situations involving long term administration of pentamidine to patients would be expected to carry a greater risk of QT prolongation and proarrhythmia compared to acute, short term treatment with the drug. The effects of pentamidine on reducing levels of HERG K$^+$ channels, while having minimal direct effects on the channel, have important implications for cardiac safety assessments conducted during drug development. Current preclinical and clinical safety studies are well positioned to detect adverse effects of drugs on cardiac repolarization following acute exposure; isolated heart experiments, for example, rapidly administer test drugs and record their electrophysiological effects over a relatively short period of time. Similarly, clinical safety studies that measure the QT interval in healthy volunteers are not designed to assess a drug's effects on the ECG over a period of time that is similar to the duration of drug therapy that may be required in a clinical setting. It is therefore possible that drugs with similar safety profiles to pentamidine (no acute effects, at clinically relevant concentrations, on the HERG K$^+$ channel and a lack of APD and QT prolongation in preclinical and clinical studies) may not be identified during drug development. Although preclinical and early clinical studies may not be able to capture QT prolonging effects of drugs due to chronic exposure, phase III clinical trials, which are typically conducted over a much longer period of time, could provide this level of information.

Drug-Induced Sodium Channel Dysfunction

The Cardiac Arrhythmia Suppression Trial (CAST) was arguably one of the first, and most important, major clinical studies to demonstrate that reduced Na^+ channel function can lead to increased mortality (CAST Investigators, 1989). The CAST trial examined the theory that the suppression of ectopic, ventricular premature complexes (defined as six or more complexes per hour) in patients with a previous myocardial infarction would reduce the risk of mortality. Post-myocardial infarction patients with either symptomatic or asymptomatic ventricular rhythm abnormalities, due to premature complexes, were randomized to receive flecainide, encainide, moricizine (all Na^+ channel-blocking, class I antiarrhythmic drugs), or placebo. Over a ten-month follow-up period since the trial's initiation, it became apparent that patients assigned to either flecainide or encainide had an increased rate of mortality (CAST Investigators, 1989). A preliminary report demonstrated that treatment with flecainide or encainide resulted in arrhythmic death or non-fatal cardiac arrest in 4.5% of drug-treated patients compared to a rate of 1.2% among patients assigned to the placebo. Additionally, the rate total mortality with flecainide or encainide was 7.7% and 3%, respectively. These devastating findings resulted in the premature termination of the CAST trial involving flecainide or encainide and the recommendation that these drugs should not be used for the treatment of ventricular arrhythmias in patients following a myocardial infarction (CAST Investigators, 1989). The part of the original study involving moricizine continued as the CAST II trial where patients that had suffered from a recent myocardial infarction (less than 90 days since the cardiac event) were randomized to moricizine or placebo; the trial was composed of an initial two-week study of moricizine 200 mg three times daily or placebo and a long term study comprising of moricizine (up to 900 mg three times daily) or placebo (CAST II Investigators, 1992). In keeping with the CAST I study, CAST II was terminated after an increased rate of death was observed in patients treated with moricizine during in the initial two-week phase of the study; 2.3% of moricizine-treated patients died compared to 0.3% of patients given a placebo (CAST II Investigators, 1992).

The CAST and CAST II trials had a profound impact on our knowledge of the mechanisms underlying ventricular arrhythmias

and optimal antiarrhythmic strategies in different patient populations. Although the antiarrhythmic drugs used in these trials did
succeed in suppressing the initial ventricular arrhythmias in patients,
they ultimately increased the rate of arrhythmic death most likely by
facilitating the formation of arrhythmogenic re-entry circuits.

Summary

Despite the fact that HERG blockade appears to be the predominant
mechanism contributing to QT prolongation and proarrhythmia,
drugs are capable of impairing repolarization and inducing arrhythmias through many other mechanisms. Alfuzosin, for example,
delays repolarization by increasing the inward Na^+ current, which
counteracts cardiac repolarization. Pentamidine, on the other hand,
acts to reduce the heart's repolarization capacity, not through direct
blockade of the HERG K^+ channel, but by causing a reduction in the
levels of the channel in cardiac myocytes. Additionally, as demonstrated by the CAST trials, QT prolongation appears to be not the
only mechanism whereby drugs may induce arrhythmias; Na^+ channel blockade in a high risk patient population proved to be a
devastating therapeutic treatment strategy. These broad ranging cellular mechanisms have important implications for how cardiac
safety is assessed during drug development; although current systems are well positioned to detect certain acute, cardiotoxic effects of
drugs, such as HERG blockade, their ability to identify drugs acting
through equally proarrhythmic mechanisms is unclear.

References

CAST II Investigators (1992). Effect of the antiarrhythmic agent moricizine
on survival after cardiac infarction. *New Engl J Med*, **327**, 227–233.
CAST Investigators (1989). Preliminary report: effect of encainide and flecainide on mortality in a randomized trial of arrhythmic suppression
after cardiac infarction. *N Engl J Med*, **321**, 406–412.
Cordes, J. *et al.* (2005). Pentamidine reduces hERG expression to prolong
the QT interval. *Br J Pharmacol*, **145**, 15–23.

Eisenhauer, M. *et al.* (1994). Incidence of cardiac arrhythmias during intravenous pentamidine therapy in HIV-infected patients. *CHEST*, **105**, 389–395.

Ficker, E. *et al.* (2004). Mechanisms of arsenic-induced prolongation of cardiac repolarization. *Mol Pharmacol*, **66**, 33–44.

Lacerda, A. *et al.* (2008). Alfuzosin delays cardiac repolarization by a novel mechanism. *J Pharmacol Exp Ther*, **324**, 427–433.

Lee, K. *et al.* (1998). Ionic mechanism of ibutilide in human atrium: evidence for a drug-induced Na+ current through a nifedipine inhibited inward channel. *J Pharmacol Exp Ther*, **286**, 9–22.

Naccarelli, G. *et al.* (1996). Electrophysiology and pharmacology of ibutilide. *Am J Cardiol*, **78**, 12–16.

Rajamani, S. *et al.* (2006). Drug-induced long QT syndrome: hERG K+ channel block and disruption of protein trafficking by fluoxetine and norfluoxetine. *Br J Pharmacol*, **149**, 481–489.

Tamargo, J. *et al.* (2004). Pharmacology of cardiac potassium channels. *Cardiovasc Res*, **62**, 9–33.

CHAPTER 6

Assessing Cardiac Safety in Drug Development

Introduction

A fundamental concept of preclinical cardiac safety studies, performed during drug development, is the use of a relatively small number of experimental systems, such as single cells, isolated cardiac tissue, isolated hearts, and *in vivo* models, to predict very rare clinical events. Preclinical safety studies provide crucial information on a drug's potential to interact with cardiac ion channels, delay repolarization, and induce cardiac arrhythmias. Clinical assessment of a drug's effects on cardiac electrophysiology, in the form of a thorough QT (TQT) study, also plays a central role in assessing the risk of drug-induced QT prolongation in large patient populations. This chapter examines international guidelines for preclinical and clinical cardiac safety assessments. In addition to describing the various preclinical models available for cardiac safety testing, and the TQT study, this chapter also explores several additional biomarkers that could be deployed in cardiac safety tests, both at the bench and bedside, to refine our ability to detect cardiotoxicity before a drug reaches the market.

Preclinical Evaluation of Cardiac Safety

A preclinical model's degree of sensitivity and specificity is central to the accurate determination of a drug's cardiac safety profile.

Sensitivity to detect potentially proarrhythmic effects of drugs is a key aspect of any preclinical model; single cell approaches that measure the HERG K$^+$ channel current can be considered to have a high level of sensitivity to detect drug blockade of the channel, however, certain isolated tissue models, and even some *in vivo* models, may fail to detect proarrhythmic effects of certain drugs. In contrast, a preclinical model with too high a level of sensitivity may yield false positive and misleading results. A preclinical model's level of specificity (i.e. its ability to accurately detect drugs with a real proarrhythmic risk) is equally important; while single cell HERG K$^+$ channel experiments can sensitively detect drug blockade of the channel, not all drugs that block the channel will have a risk of inducing arrhythmias in humans.

In addition to determining a drug's cardiac safety profile and its proarrhythmic potential, preclinical models can also provide insight into a drug's safety margin by studying a drug's effects using a range of different concentrations. The safety margin can be defined as the difference between the therapeutic concentration of a drug and the concentration that yields the maximal effects on cardiac electrophysiological parameters. The greater the safety margin of a drug, the lower is its risk of inducing adverse events in clinical situations in which the drug's concentration may become elevated, for example in the setting of disease-induced hepatic impairment or co-administration of drugs with similar metabolic pathways. Assessing the cardiovascular effects of new drugs in various preclinical systems is currently recommended by regulatory authorities based on the International Conference of Harmonization (ICH) topic S7B guidance document. In the following sections, the ICH S7B guidelines and the benefits and limitations of several major preclinical cardiac safety platforms, used during drug development, are discussed.

The ICH S7B Guidelines

The ICH S7B guidelines (The Non-Clinical Evaluation of the Potential for Delayed Ventricular Repolarization (QT

Prolongation) by Human Pharmaceuticals, S7B, ICH, 2005a) provide a series of recommendations for drug developers to test an
early-stage drug in preclinical experiments to determine its potential to impair repolarization and induce QT prolongation. Tests
recommended by ICH S7B help to ascertain a dose-response profile of a drug, and its metabolites, for prolonging repolarization
and, when combined with additional information, results from
these studies are used to carefully evaluate a drug's safety profile.
Importantly, the ICH S7B guidelines recommend conducting preclinical cardiac safety experiments before the initiation of a drug's
clinical development as information from preclinical cardiac safety
studies can help guide a drug's clinical development. The preclinical cardiac safety strategy recommended by the ICH S7B guidelines
is depicted in Figure 1.

At the very core of the ICH S7B guidelines is the recommendation to test the ability of drugs to directly block the HERG K$^+$
channel, using a cellular assay, and to induce QT prolongation in
in vivo animal models. The guidelines state that, as cellular measurements of the HERG K$^+$ channel current and QT measurements are
complementary to one another, drugs should be evaluated in both
types of experiment. Another important aspect of the preclinical testing strategy described in the ICH S7B guidelines is the use of
reference drugs that are known to induce QT prolongation in
humans; a reference drug acts as a vital benchmark to determine a
test drug's cardiac safety profile. Additionally, the use of a reference
drug can also validate a model's sensitivity and specificity for

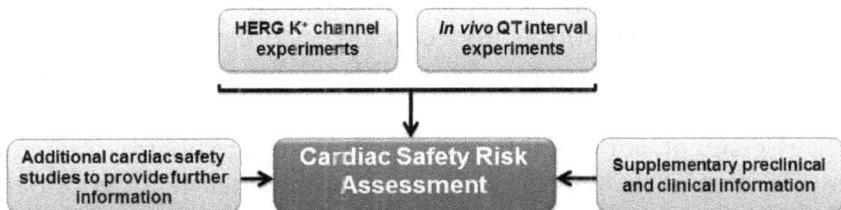

Figure 1: The components comprising integrated preclinical cardiac risk
assessments, according to ICH S7B guidelines.

detecting drug-induced QT prolongation and proarrhythmia. The ICH S7B guidelines suggest, when possible, using reference drugs belonging to the same chemical or pharmacological class as the test drug; for example, if a new antiarrhythmic drug has a similar mode of action, and chemical structure, as dofetilide (a Class III antiarrhythmic that intentionally blocks the HERG K^+ channel, and is associated with a risk of QT prolongation) it would be prudent to consider using dofetilde as the reference drug.

In addition to the HERG K^+ channel and *in vivo* studies recommended by the ICH S7B guidelines, further preclinical safety studies are suggested to provide a greater understanding of a drug's safety profile and its potential to induce repolarization abnormalities in humans. Such follow-up studies are recommended when results differ between the two core preclinical studies, or if clinical data highlights a potential safety signal. For example if a test drug has not been shown to reduce the HERG K^+ channel current in the cellular study but it goes on to induce QT prolongation in *in vivo* experiments, the drug's safety profile could be further evaluated in additional preclinical models, or using different experimental designs, to help identify the cause of these discordant safety findings.

The final stage of the ICH S7B-recommended preclinical safety strategy is the integration of data generated to assess a drug's overall cardiac safety profile and evaluate its risk of inducing QT prolongation in humans. A number of factors that should be considered at this stage include the relationship between the drug concentrations required to induce HERG K^+ channel blockade or QT prolongation *in vivo* and those needed to elicit the drug's desired therapeutic effects (the safety margin). It is also important to compare the drug's effects on repolarization to those of reference drugs. Leveraging additional information from studies outside of those recommended by the ICH S7B guidelines also forms a central component of a drug's risk assessment. For example knowledge of a drug's pharmacokinetic profile, such as its half-life, could help in the interpretation of data from *in vivo* safety studies.

In the following sections, the strengths and weaknesses of a variety of currently used preclinical models are discussed.

Single Cell Safety Studies

Cell based systems remain an important component of preclinical drug safety testing; their relatively low cost and high throughput capabilities make them an attractive assay to include in the drug development process. A number of different single cell tests have been developed to detect the ability of drugs to prolong the QT interval in humans.

Radioligand binding assays, still used extensively in drug discovery, were previously used to determine the ability of drugs to bind to HERG K$^+$ channels. However, measurements of drug binding to the HERG K$^+$ channel provide no indication of how the drug can alter the channel's function. Additionally, ion channels are not static proteins that exist in a single state within the cell membrane. Membrane depolarization significantly alters the conformation of the ion channel protein which in turn opens the channel's pore, permitting the flow of ions. These structural changes can significantly alter the ability of drugs to bind to, and block, the HERG channel. With this in mind, measuring drug binding to HERG K$^+$ channels, using electrically quiescent cells, has significant limitations. For these reasons, this assay is no longer recommended by regulatory authorities.

Measurements of HERG K$^+$ channel currents in single cells are considered to be one of the most powerful ways of predicting a drug's proarrhythmic liability. Isolating native myocytes from the intact heart is costly, time consuming and technically difficult, therefore HERG K$^+$ channel measurements are predominantly performed in mammalian cell lines that artificially overexpress the ion channel. Traditionally these experiments, although powerful, were limited by their labour intensive and low throughput nature. However, in recent years medium to high throughput systems have been developed, such as the IonWorks and QPatch systems.

Studies have attempted to measure the degree of HERG K$^+$ channel blockade and correlate this with a risk of QT prolongation and arrhythmias. Extrapolating HERG K$^+$ channel data to the animal or human levels is fraught with difficulty, and HERG blockade is widely regarded as only one part of the complex puzzle of drug-induced QT prolongation and proarrhythmia.

HERG experiments are only capable of detecting agents that can acutely alter the ion channel's function. However, a number of drugs that possess multi ion channel blocking effects have been reported, with notable examples being verapamil, amiodarone and ranalozine. As such drugs block the HERG K^+ channel one could assume that these agents cause QT prolongation and pose a risk of inducing arrhythmias in patients; however, this does not appear to be the case. Verapamil is known for its L-type Ca^{2+} channel blocking effects which appear to counteract its HERG effects and result in no proarrhythmic risk. Similarly, amiodarone blocks a range of cardiac ion channels and studies have shown that it induces QT prolongation; however, owing to amiodarone's homogenous effects on cardiac repolarization (it does not significantly alter the repolarization gradient) it poses no significant risk of proarrhythmia. In both of these examples, measurement of HERG K^+ currents alone would yield misleading results. It is therefore prudent to screen new drugs against a variety of cardiac ion channels to more accurately gauge their safety profiles.

The Purkinje Fiber Model

The Purkinje fiber model is commonly used in preclinical cardiac safety screening and it has a number of advantages over single cell approaches; this model can be used to record changes in APD and morphology. Purkinje fibers are also capable of recording arrhythmogenic phenomena such as EADs and triggered activity, which further validate its use for cardiac safety testing.

However, the Purkinje fiber model has several important limitations, perhaps the most significant being reports of sharply contrasting effects of drugs in Purkinje fibers compared to other preclinical models. For example, dronedarone has been shown to shorten repolarization times in the Purkinje fiber but induce APD prolongation in ventricular muscle preparations (Varró *et al.*, 2001). Additionally terfenadine, which is known to prolong the AP in isolated heart preparations, only minimally prolonged repolarization times in canine Purkinje fibers (Gintant *et al.*, 2001). There are also significant species-related differences in the response of Purkinje fibers to QT prolonging drugs; studying a drug's effects in Purkinje fibers from certain species could result in false negative drug safety data.

Additionally, when testing the effects of drugs on APD in Purkinje fibers, a wide range of concentrations should be used to examine bimodal ion channel effects. A low concentration of a drug, for example, may block the HERG K^+ channel alone and cause significant APD prolongation; higher drug concentrations could also exert effects on other channels, such as the L-type Ca^{2+} channel, which could counteract the HERG blockade.

Purkinje fibers also have the potential to be overly sensitive to drug-induced delays in repolarization and they could inappropriately generate false positive data by significantly amplifying a drug's effects. This attribute of the Purkinje fiber model results from its isolation and separation from ventricular tissue; ordinarily, Purkinje fibers are electrically coupled to ventricular tissue which likely acts to reduce repolarization times in the *in situ* Purkinje fiber. Additionally, once Purkinje fibers are immediately isolated from the heart, they are electrically unstable and require stabilization for a 60- to 90-minute period before drug experiments should be conducted. Finally, although Purkinje fibers can detect APD prolongation, EADs, and other arrhythmogenic signals, they are unable to detect changes in repolarization gradients which have been shown to play a central role in the generation of drug-induced arrhythmias.

The Ventricular Wedge Model

The ventricular wedge model has been successfully used to examine some of the fundamental mechanisms underlying drug-induced arrhythmias. Using the ventricular wedge model and a range of pharmacological agents, research groups have been able to create surrogate models of congenital long QT syndrome and powerful systems in which to determine a drug's cardiac safety profile.

The ventricular wedge model involves dissecting a wedge of tissue from the left ventricular free wall, often from the canine or rabbit heart, and perfusing it via a coronary artery. Electrodes are then inserted into multiple regions of the ventricular wedge to simultaneously record APs from epicardial, endocardial and mid myocardial (M-cell) layers which permit the measurement of the transmural dispersion of repolarization (TDR). The electrophysiological differences between these three areas of the ventricle underlies the TDR theory of arrhythmogenesis; excessive prolongation of APs in the M-cell layer in response to HERG blocking drugs creates discrete zones of refractory tissue around which stimuli from neighboring regions are forced to circumvent, establishing arrhythmogenic re-entrant circuits. For more information on arrhythmia mechanisms that have been identified through the use of the ventricular wedge model see Chapter 4.

By combining APD measurements with transmural ECG recordings, correlations between TDR and T-wave parameters have also been proposed. Increases in TDR have been shown to induce large changes in the interval between the peak and the end of the T-wave ($T_{peak} - T_{end}$). However, ECG recordings performed in the ventricular wedge model do not correspond well to clinical ECG recordings. Only two ECG electrodes are used in wedge experiments, across a very small sample of tissue encompassing only the thickness of the ventricular wall. While TDR does appear to correspond to $T_{peak} - T_{end}$ measurements in the ventricular wedge model, other gradients of repolarization, which have also been shown to play a pivotal role in arrhythmogenesis exist in the intact heart. True clinical ECG recordings take into account the electrical activity of the entire myocardium, not just one small section. Indeed, findings from the intact heart suggest that $T_{peak} - T_{end}$ measurements could be reflective of the global dispersion of repolarization; encompassing a range of repolarization gradients. The potential for $T_{peak} - T_{end}$ measurements to act as a cardiac safety biomarker is discussed later in this chapter.

Isolated Heart Models

The isolated heart model has been successfully used to provide important information on the mechanisms that give rise to arrhythmias.

A wealth of electrophysiological data can be obtained from an iso-lated, beating heart including, measurements of APD, repolarization heterogeneity and heart rate. Single cell studies, for all their advantages in terms of throughput and the depth of electrophysiological data at the ion channel level that can be obtained, cannot clarify the precise relationship between impaired repolarization and EADs at the single cell level and arrhythmias at the whole heart level. Furthermore, single cell studies fail to take into consideration the regional differences in cardiac electrophysiology that are present in the heart. Whole heart experiments contain the full complement of cardiac myocytes that are electrically coupled to one another in their native environment. Unlike single cell cardiac safety experiments, whole heart preparations can detect and measure drug-induced alterations in repolarization gradients.

The perfused heart model has been successfully used for both the study of arrhythmia mechanisms and preclinical cardiac safety assessments of drugs. Following the rapid removal and perfusion of the heart, it regains a healthy coloration and it begins contracting rhythmically. Figure 2 illustrates the experimental setup of the

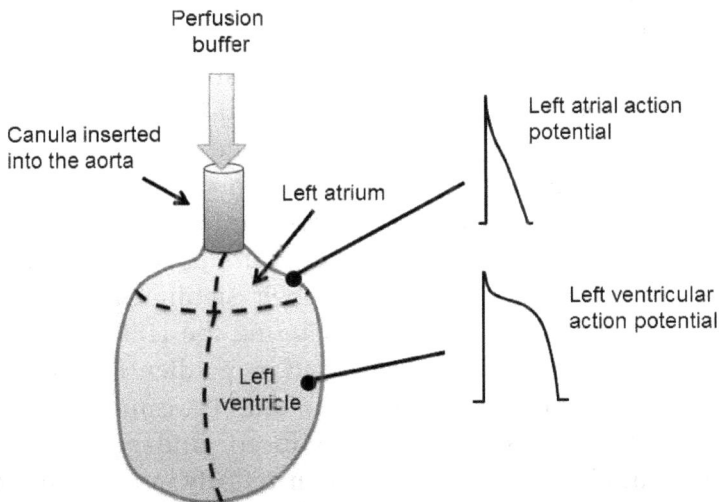

Figure 2: The isolated heart experimental setup.

isolated heart model in which a cannula inserted into the aorta perfuses the heart with a physiological solution and electrodes placed on the atria and ventricles record electrical activity.

In keeping with other animal tissue models, including the ventricular wedge preparation, another major advantage of using isolated hearts in preclinical safety studies is the ability to mimic a number of different clinical scenarios that are known to increase the risk of drug-induced arrhythmias. By administering a drug and controlling the heart rate using, artificial pacing, for example, one can recapitulate a number of clinical settings that may increase the risk of arrhythmias.

In Vivo Models

Various *in vivo* models are currently used by the pharmaceutical industry for cardiac safety testing; these have several advantages over isolated heart preparations. Perhaps one of the major advantages of *in vivo* models is their ability to closely mimic a biological environment that is comparable to that seen in humans; for example, the influence of drug metabolism and polypharmacy upon a test compound's effects on the heart can be accurately determined using an *in vivo* model. Additionally, *in vivo* models preserve the autonomic nervous system's innervations of the heart; stimulation of the autonomic nervous system can induce significant changes in ventricular repolarization gradients (Mantravadi *et al.*, 2007).

The use of anesthesia is a common approach when assessing a drug's cardiac safety profile in an *in vivo* model, however, the use of anesthesia has some major drawbacks. Perhaps the greatest limitation associated with anesthetics is their significant effects on a number of cardiac ion channels, including the HERG K^+ channel, which could alter cardiac repolarization gradients and generate potentially misleading safety information. Transmural repolarization gradients are significantly reduced under pentobarbital anesthesia and it becomes difficult to artificially induce arrhythmias (Antzelevitch *et al.*, 2001). Additionally, pentobarbital and isoflurane anesthesia have been shown to exert notable antiarrhythmic effects in the presence of quinidine and astemizole (Yamamoto *et al.*, 2001). When using an *in vivo* model in conjunction with pentobarbital anesthesia experimental maneuvers in addition to HERG K$^+$ channel blockade may be required to induce arrhythmias; when using pentobarbital anesthesia in guinea pig or rabbit models, for example, co-administration of adrenaline or phenylephrine is required to induce arrhythmias (Farkas *et al.*, 2008; Michael *et al.*, 2008). Such experimental maneuvers question the validity of using these models for cardiac safety testing. Despite these limitations, *in vivo* models, even in the presence of an anesthetic agent, can provide key insight into a drug's potentially proarrhythmic effects in human patients; measuring various ECG parameters, such as the QT interval, can help to determine a drug's effects on cardiac electrophysiology.

To increase the predictive power of *in vivo* cardiac safety approaches, a drug's effects could be studied in a model that mimics several aspects of specific patient populations, who are more vulnerable to drug-induced cardiac toxicity. One such preclinical system is the canine model with chronic atrioventricular (AV) block; as discussed in Chapter 2, the AV node ordinarily controls the transmission of electrical impulses from the atria to the ventricles. In this model, a surgical procedure is used to severely damage the AV node and prevent the conduction of all of the atrial impulses to the ventricles — this impairment of cardiac conduction results in a state of bradycardia, in which the heart rate is significantly reduced, and the gradual development of bradycardia-induced heart failure. Once AV block has been established, and bradycardia-induced heart failure develops, a series of pathophysiological events take place over a period of two to four weeks in which the heart's electrical and structural attributes are substantially remodeled in an attempt to compensate for the bradycardia. Cardiac remodeling that takes places includes myocardial hypertrophy, reductions in the heart's repolarization capacity through the down-regulation of K$^+$ channels, raised levels of sympathetic drive to the heart, and increased levels of angiotensin II (Sugiyama *et al.*, 2008). Importantly these processes are likely to increase the risk of drug-induced QT prolongation and arrhythmias and thus establish a preclinical safety model that is sensitized to detect drug-induced proarrhythmia. Studies with drugs known to induce arrhythmias have confirmed the sensitivity of the AV block canine model. Although administration of a cardiotoxic drug readily induces triggered activity in the canine AV block model in the first two weeks, ventricular arrhythmias are rarely observed; however, when the same drug is given four weeks after the induction of AV block (once cardiac remodeling has taken place), arrhythmias are often recorded (Sugiyama *et al.*, 2008).

The validity of studying the cardiac effects of all new drugs in a system which models a high risk patient population remains debatable as the increased sensitivity of the model could generate false positive results. Nevertheless, as discussed in Chapter 9, drug safety testing in a specific animal model of human disease could yield vital safety information, particularly for drugs whose intended patients are commonly afflicted with the same comorbidity.

The relative strengths and weaknesses of several leading preclinical cardiac safety models are summarized in Figures 3 and 4. Figure 3 scores the throughput of different models against the arrhythmogenic signal that can be recorded from the model. Single cell HERG experiments, for example, can be performed at a medium to high throughput rate, however, only ion channel data can be obtained

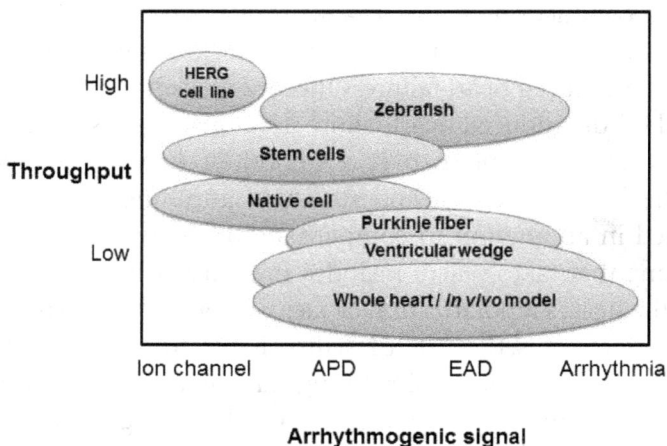

Figure 3:   A competitive assessment of leading preclinical cardiac safety systems.

Preclinical model attributes

Mammalian
cell line

- Artificial over expression of human ion channels
- HERG K⁺ channel recordings can be obtained

Native
myocytes

- Contain full complement of ion channels and intracellular proteins
- Single ion channel measurements
- Action potential recordings
- EADs, DADs, and single cell arrhythmias

Increasing
physiological
complexity

Ventricular
wedge

- Captures cardiac electrical heterogeneity
- Can record action potentials from different regions, surrogate QT measurements
- Can detect different arrhythmogenic mechanisms (re-entry, EADs, DADs)
- Clinically-relevant arrhythmias can be induced and recorded

Isolated
perfused
heart

- Isolated, working heart
- Action potentials and ECGs can be recorded
- Multiple arrhythmia mechanisms can be recorded
- Clinically-relevant arrhythmias can be induced and recorded

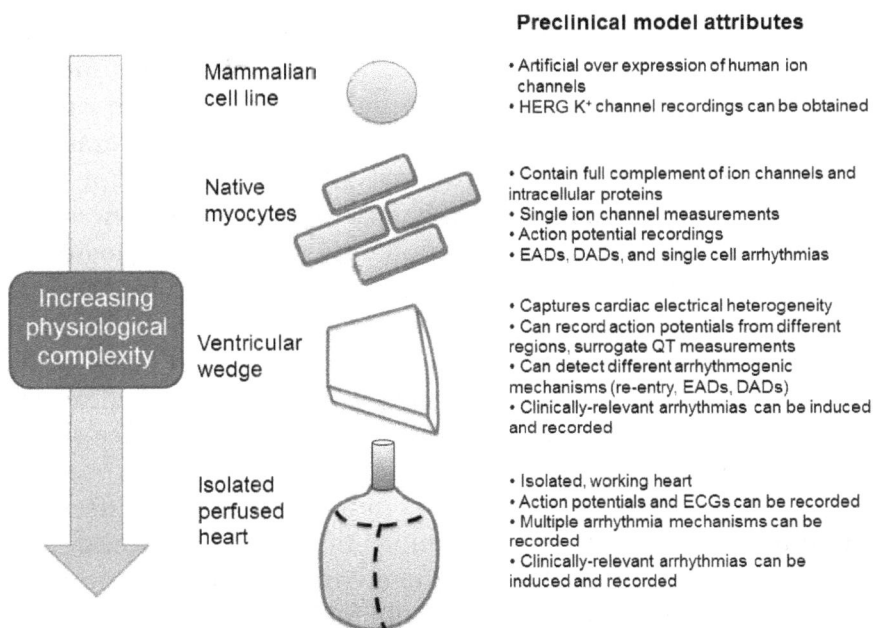

Figure 4:   The key attributes of leading preclinical cardiac safety systems.

from this system. In contrast, whole heart or *in vivo* experiments can capture a wide array of potential proarrhythmia signals from APD and QT prolongation through to EADs and arrhythmias, however, these models suffer from a low throughput. From a theoretical standpoint, a position within the upper right quadrant of this matrix would signal a preclinical model in which proarrhythmic effects of drugs could be recorded at a high throughput. Figure 4 describes several of the main attributes for currently-used preclinical models.

The Impact of Species-Related Differences in Cardiac Electrophysiology on Preclinical Drug Safety Assessment

Major differences exist in the cardiac electrophysiological profiles of different animal species that may be used for preclinical safety testing. Safety studies have used isolated hearts from a range of species, including canine, rabbit, guinea pig, and mouse. Importantly there are several species-related differences in cardiac electrophysiology between these models; mouse hearts, for example, have triangular APs and rely less on the HERG K^+ channel for repolarization, while guinea pig hearts lack the transient outward K^+ current seen in other species. Additionally, identical physiological or pharmacological maneuvers can yield contrasting results; whereas hypokalemia is extremely proarrhythmic in the mouse heart, it appears to be only mildly proarrhythmic in the rabbit heart, while arrhythmias cannot be recorded in the isolated guinea pig heart. As a result of these differences, great care needs to be taken when selecting a particular species for preclinical cardiac safety testing.

One of the most revealing studies into species-related differences in cardiac electrophysiology determined the effects of dofetilide and quinidine, both QT prolonging drugs, on APs recorded from six different animal species (Lu *et al.*, 2001). Upon isolation and stabilization of rabbit, canine, guinea pig, swine, goat, and sheep Purkinje fibers, dofetilide was infused for up to 25 minutes and effects of the drug on the APD were measured. The relative change in APD seen was remarkably different across the six species. Rabbit Purkinje fibers appeared to be the most sensitive to dofetilde; in this species the APD was significantly increased from 189 to 655 ms. Notable APD prolongation was also recorded in canine and goat Purkinje fibers exposed to dofetilide, although the magnitude of APD change was less than that recorded in rabbit Purkinje fibers (65% and 61% change in APD, respectively) (Lu *et al.*, 2001). The effects of dofetilide in the swine and sheep Purkinje fibers were, however, considerably more modest; APD increased by only 18% and 30%, respectively. Additionally, dofetilide failed to significantly increase APD in guinea pig Purkinje fibers, in contrast to findings from all Purkinje fibers from other species (Lu *et al.*, 2001). Major differences in the effects quinidine on the Purkinje fiber APD were also seen across the six species; after 20 minutes, quinidine induced significant prolongation of APD in rabbit and canine Purkinje fibers, it had no effect on APD in guinea pig, swine, and goat Purkinje fibers, and it significantly reduced APD in sheep Purkinje fibers (Lu *et al.*, 2001). In a final series of experiments, the proarrhythmic effects of dofetilide and quinidine were examined in Purkinje fibers; although the drugs evoked EADs in 89% and 91% of rabbit Purkinje fibers, respectively, EADs were not observed in Purkinje fibers from any other species, despite significant APD prolongation (Lu *et al.*, 2001).

This study has several important implications for preclinical drug safety testing. Firstly, large discrepancies in the observed effects of drugs, known to induce QT prolongation and arrhythmias, across different species emphasize the need for careful selection of species for preclinical safety testing. Secondly, the demonstration of significant APD prolongation in rabbit, canine, swine, goat, and sheep Purkinje fibers yet the appearance of EADs in only rabbit preparations demonstrates the fact that measurements of APD alone may be relatively poor predictors of drug-induced arrhythmia risk. The potential for a drug to induce other proarrhythmic effects, including EADs, triggered activity, and changes in repolarization gradients, in a range of different models, must be incorporated into preclinical safety assessments in order to accurately determine cardiac safety.

Methods to Provoke Arrhythmias in Preclinical Studies

Programmed electrical stimulation

A common technique used in cardiac tissue, whole heart, and *in vivo* animal preparations involves the application of artificial premature stimuli to provoke arrhythmias — this methodology is called programmed electrical stimulation (PES). In a PES protocol a train of paced stimuli are delivered to the heart and the last stimulus is gradually applied closer to the preceding stimulus. For example, if a heart is to be paced at a cycle length of 200 ms (every 200 ms a single stimulus will be applied to the preparation), the last stimulus of the first PES cycle will be delivered at the standard 200 ms interval. However, the second PES cycle will deliver the last stimulus at a 199 ms interval; this cycle will repeat itself whereby the last stimulus

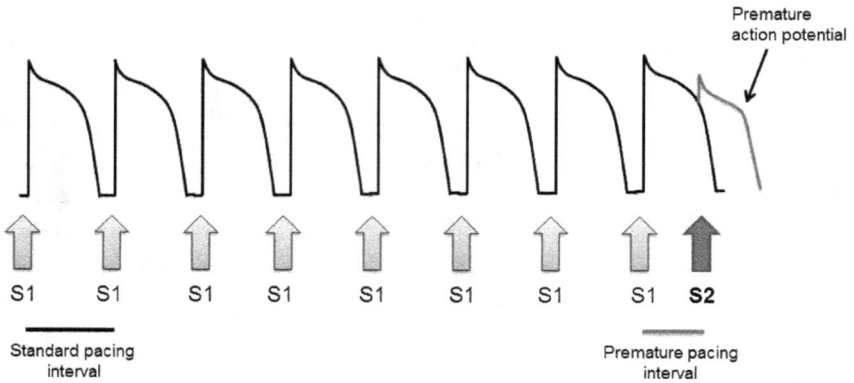

Figure 5:   Action potential recordings during a programmed electrical stimulation cycle.

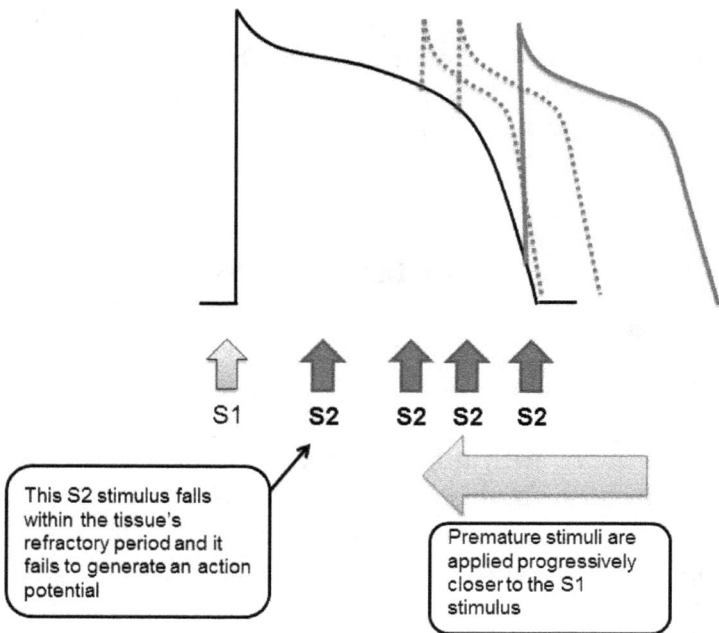

Figure 6:   Premature action potentials generated during programmed electrical stimulation.

is applied increasingly closer to its preceding stimulus. In PES protocols the train of standard stimuli are often referred to as S1 stimuli and the prematurely delivered stimuli are known as S2 stimuli — APs are generated following both S1 and S2 stimuli (Figure 5). Eventually a premature stimulation will be delivered too close to the preceding stimulus resulting in no AP generated — this point reflects the tissue's refractory period where the cardiac tissue has not yet sufficiently recovered from the original excitation of the preceding stimulus (Figure 6).

As discussed in Chapter 4, a common cause of ventricular arrhythmias is a triggering event, such as an EAD, which takes place during the repolarization phase. PES protocols, by applying premature stimulations during the repolarization period, therefore mimic EADs, and are powerful tools to provoke arrhythmias in preclinical preparations.

Reductions in the extracellular K^+ concentration

Another common maneuver that is used to assess a drug's potential for inducing cardiac arrhythmias is to lower the concentration of K^+ in the solution used to perfuse the tissue. After the induction of hypokalemia, by lowering the K^+ concentration, experimental tissues become sensitized to drug-induced arrhythmias; a number of preclinical studies have described how administration of a drug known to block the HERG K^+ channel fails to produce arrhythmias on its own, however, subsequent lowering of the K^+ concentration reproducibly leads to ventricular arrhythmias (Milberg *et al.*, 2002). Initially, low K^+ solutions were considered to exert their effects solely through direct interaction with the HERG K^+ channel. However, more recently a series of experiments have revealed that hypokalemic solutions reduce additional repolarizing ion channel currents (Killeen *et al.*, 2007). In isolated ventricular myocytes, hypokalemic solutions evoked significant reductions in I_{to} and I_{K1} K^+ channel currents. Additionally, in isolated heart experiments, hypokalemic solutions increased the ventricular APD and altered the ventricular repolarization gradient (Killeen *et al.*, 2007).

The use of hypokalemic solutions to provoke drug-induced ventricular arrhythmias has a number of advantages. Firstly, the use of low K^+ solutions in conjunction with HERG blocking agents to generate arrhythmias correlates with several clinical reports describing drug-induced QT prolongation and arrhythmias in patients with hypokalemia. Additionally, as hypokalemic solutions specifically target and impair cardiac repolarization they could model the effects of a drug in high risk patients that have a reduced repolarization capacity. Finally, the use of hypokalemic solutions avoids the use of additional drugs to provoke arrhythmias; such drugs may have effects on a wide array of other ion channel currents and internal signaling pathways.

Nevertheless, despite these advantages there is a risk of falsely identifying drugs with a proarrhythmia risk when using hypokalemic solutions in drug safety studies. In the setting of hypokalemia, major reductions in the extracellular K^+ concentration could overly sensitize the animal model to drug-induced proarrhythmia and generate false positive data. Additionally, cardiac safety data obtained for a range of drug doses in the setting of hypokalemia would need to be interpreted with great caution. For example, testing a drug's proarrhythmic potential, in the presence of hypokalemic solutions, using a series of increasing doses would be expected to result in a much smaller safety margin compared to studying the same doses in the absence of hypokalemic solutions.

Clinical Evaluation of Cardiac Safety

The Thorough QT study

Following several reports of proarrhythmia associated with non-cardiovascular medications, global regulators responded by designing and implementing a range of preclinical and clinical guidelines that provide advice for developers to study a drug's potential to delay repolarization and increase the risk of ventricular arrhythmias. The ICH Topic E14 guidelines (ICH E14), entitled "The Clinical Evaluation of QT/QTc Interval Prolongation and

Proarrhythmic Potential for Non-Antiarrhythmic Drugs," were published in November 2005 and they represented an important milestone in drug safety assessment (ICH, 2005b). Briefly, the purpose of the ICH E14 guidelines is to provide a methodology for assessing the effects of drugs on cardiac repolarization parameters by closely monitoring the QT interval in healthy volunteers (in certain circumstances other patient populations may be studied) following drug administration. These human clinical studies are referred to as Thorough QT (TQT) studies. The ICH E14 guidelines issued by the International Conference on Harmonization, on behalf of major global regulatory bodies, provided in depth guidance for how these studies should be conducted and outlined the potential implications for drugs demonstrating significant QT prolongation.

TQT studies have now become a standard feature of drug development. The ICH E14 guidelines state that TQT studies should investigate drugs at two different doses — a dose expected to be used in the clinic, should the drug be approved, to achieve the desired effect, and a supratherapeutic dose of the drug. This latter dose allows developers to assess the drug's effect on the QT interval in situations in which the drug may reach higher than anticipated concentrations in the body; impaired drug metabolism due to concomitant medication use or disease, for example, could substantially raise the drug's concentration which may lead to toxic effects on the heart.

Thorough QT study design

The overarching aim of a TQT study is to detect, with a relative degree of sensitivity, the ability of a drug to prolong the QT interval in healthy volunteers. Eliminating the risk of detecting QT prolongation in patients due to factors other than the study drug is therefore an important consideration in the design of these studies and appropriate patient selection accordingly plays a central role in a TQT study; typical exclusion criteria would include patients with QT prolongation greater than 450 ms prior to drug administration, concomitant medications that could increase the risk of QT prolongation, and other patient characteristics/disease states such as congenital long QT syndrome or hypokalemia.

Results from TQT studies are used to ascertain the risk of QT prolongation in the drug's target patient population and to assess the need for further cardiac monitoring during the drug's future clinical development. For example, if a drug is shown to induce mean QT prolongation of 5 ms or more in a TQT study, its developers would be expected to conduct extensive ECG monitoring in future clinical trials; in particular, developers would be expected to record ECGs in patients at times in which the drug is expected to reach peak plasma concentrations and to closely track adverse events in specific patient subpopulations such as those with heart failure, an impaired capacity for drug metabolism, and in patients presenting with electrolyte abnormalities. Therefore, developers of drugs that have been shown to induce a mean QT prolongation of 5 ms or more in a TQT study would be expected to incur substantial costs due to these additional monitoring requirements in subsequent clinical trials.

A fundamental aspect of a TQT study is the use of a positive control drug, known to induce QT prolongation, to ensure the test's sensitivity to detect relatively small changes in a patient's QT interval. Moxifloxacin is used as the positive control drug in TQT studies as it readily induces QT prolongation in healthy volunteers (by approximately 5–10 ms). The ICH E14 guidelines state that in certain cases, the positive control drug used in a TQT study could belong to the same class as the test drug if its effects on prolonging the QT interval have already been established. The ability to record the QT prolonging effects of the positive control drug validates the TQT study's sensitivity to detect small changes in the QT interval following administration of the study drug.

TQT studies have typically enrolled 100–300 healthy volunteers who are randomized to receive either the study drug or positive control. In order to reduce their size and cost, a crossover design approach to the trial can be considered in which test subjects are administered, at different points in time, both the test and positive control drug. For example, if both of the drugs have relatively short half lives, switching patients from one therapy to another after a short period of time would be feasible. However, if the test drug has a slow onset of action, such crossover trial designs are not appropriate and a conventional parallel group TQT study should be conducted.

An additional principle of a TQT study is to evaluate the pathophysiological consequences of drug concentrations that are considerably higher than those required to elicit a therapeutic response. These requirements likely stem from initial observations of drug-induced cardiac toxicity with terfenadine and ketoconazole co-therapy. Therefore, if possible, a TQT study should administer the test drug at both therapeutic and supratherapeutic doses to explore for an effect on the QT interval. However, in many cases the use of a supratherapeutic drug dose may not be possible due to other adverse events or issues regarding the drug's tolerability. In some cases, a drug's mode of action and its desired therapeutic effects could preclude the use of a supratherapeutic dose; administration of a supratherapeutic dose of an insulin-like drug for the treatment of type II diabetes, for example, could lead to major adverse events such as life-threatening hypoglycemia. The ICH E14 guidelines also state that another approach to study the effects of high test drug concentrations would be to inhibit a drug's hepatic metabolism.

The precise timing of a drug's TQT study is an important consideration for developers. Due to the TQT study's design, thorough knowledge of a drug's pharmacokinetic and pharmacodynamic effects would be required which precludes the initiation of such a study prior to a Phase I clinical trial. However, due to the substantial cost of conducting a TQT study a developer may wait until proof-of-concept Phase II efficacy data in a drug's target patient population are seen. Late conduct of a TQT study can have important consequences for a developer and may even lead to a delay in a drug's launch. In October 2010 the FDA issued a complete response letter for extended-release exenatide for the treatment of type II diabetes; the FDA requested that a TQT study of the drug should be performed. In addition to other requests from the FDA, the need to conduct a TQT study for the drug, coupled with the time required for the agency to review these new data, had been estimated to delay the drug's launch by at least one year. Despite the prior approval, and current use, of exenatide for type II diabetes, the reformulation of the drug to permit longer dosing intervals (through the use of high dose of exenatide administered subcutaneously) could potentially result in exposure to significantly higher concentrations of the drug. Indeed, the ICH E14 guidelines state that a TQT study would not only be required for new chemical entities seeking approval, but also for new doses or routes of administration of currently available medications that would be expected to lead to higher plasma concentrations of the drug. Additionally, TQT studies could also be requested by regulatory agencies if a licensed drug is seeking approval for use in a new patient population or for a new therapeutic indication. As we will examine later on in this chapter, TQT studies may even be requested for previously approved drugs following reports of cardiac toxicity in patients.

Additional Biomarkers to Detect Drug-Induced Proarrhythmia

Although measurements of QT prolongation, and associated reports of ventricular arrhythmias, have provided evidence in support of QT measurements to predict drug-induced proarrhythmia, the QT interval appears to be an imperfect marker of arrhythmia risk. For example, although excessive drug-induced QT prolongation is accepted to pose a major risk of proarrhythmia and sudden cardiac death, the precise relationship between more subtle increases in the QT interval and arrhythmias is less clear. Additionally several drugs, such as amiodarone and ranolazine, that are capable of inducing QT prolongation in patients have remarkably strong cardiac safety profiles. With these considerations in mind, clinical studies have attempted to identify additional biomarkers of drug-induced proarrhythmia that have the potential to be incorporated into routine clinical safety evaluations. Among the most promising novel biomarkers are short term variability of repolarization, T wave morphology changes, and measurements of the $T_{peak}-T_{end}$ interval. Each of these biomarkers are discussed below.

Variability of repolarization

Several studies have suggested that the variability of repolarization parameters, such as the APD or QT interval, are accurate predictors of drug-induced proarrhythmia. Hinterseer and colleagues (2008) tested the hypothesis that patients at risk of drug-induced QT prolongation and ventricular arrhythmias had measureable differences in the short term variability (STV) of their QT intervals compared to healthy volunteers.

ECGs from patients who had prior documented episodes of drug-induced torsade de pointes (TdP) were compared with those obtained from control individuals and various parameters were assessed, including the QT interval, RR interval, and QRS durations. Patients with a history of TdP presented with significantly greater levels of STV of the QT interval compared to control individuals (8.1 versus 3.6 ms, P < 0.001). In fact, STV of the QT interval was the only parameter that was significantly different between these two subgroups of patients; QT, QRS, and RR intervals were comparable (Hinterseer *et al.*, 2008). An additional clinical study supports these findings. In patients administered sotalol, the STV of the QT interval transiently increased from a baseline value of 6.9 to 12.2 ms prior to the initiation of TdP (Kaab *et al.*, 2003). Collectively, these results suggest that patients at risk of developing drug-induced proarrhythmia can be identified on the basis of a latent repolarization abnormality that is present prior to the administration of a drug.

Preclinical studies also support the concept of repolarization variability as a predictor of drug-induced proarrhythmia. *In vivo* findings from anesthetized dogs with chronic AV block, demonstrated that sertindole (an anti-psychotic drug) at both low and high doses induced significant QT prolongation and TdP (Thomsen *et al.*, 2006). However, both doses of the drug significantly prolonged the QT interval, whereas only the higher dose actually induced arrhythmias. The authors of this study measured APDs recorded from the endocardial wall of the left ventricle and showed that animals administered the high dose of sertindole exhibited a significant increase in the STV of APD (Thomsen *et al.*, 2006). Therefore in keeping with the above clinical studies, measurement of repolarization STV was the only parameter that could successfully predict drug-induced proarrhythmia. These findings were further advanced by the use of concurrent drugs to yield antiarrhythmic effects and prevent sertindole-induced arrhythmias. Levcromakalim, a K^+ channel activator, was given to sertindole-treated animals to explore for changes in the QT interval and STV of APD. Intriguingly, one dose of levcromakalim significantly reduced the frequency of TdP episodes without any effect on the QT interval; however, STV of APD was significantly reduced (Thomsen *et al.*, 2006). These findings further demonstrate the intricate relationship between repolarization STV and drug-induced proarrhythmia.

Variability of repolarization, coupled with additional biomarkers, has been successfully used to predict the proarrhythmic potential of drugs in preclinical cardiac safety models (Hondeghem *et al.*, 2001). An important study assessed the effects of over 700 drugs on the morphology of ventricular APs recorded from isolated hearts; drug-induced arrhythmias were often preceded by repolarization instability and changes to the morphology of the AP (it became triangulated in shape) (Hondeghem *et al.*, 2001). (Figure 7 illustrates proarrhythmic AP triangulation.) In particular, drugs with proarrhythmic effects evoked APD prolongation, instability, and AP triangulation; in contrast, in the absence of triangulation and repolarization instability, AP prolongation failed to evoke arrhythmias

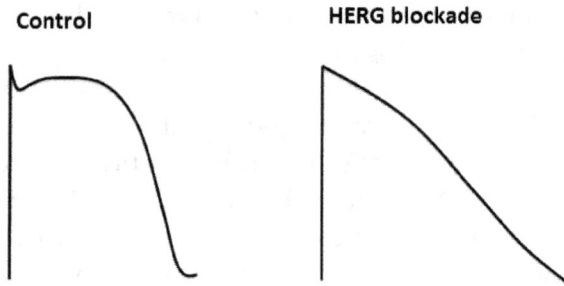

Figure 7: Ventricular action potential triangulation induced by HERG blockade.

(Hondeghem *et al.*, 2001) These findings demonstrate that such additional biomarkers have the potential to yield a more sophisticated assessment of a drug's cardiac safety profile. Combining measurements of AP triangulation, reverse-use dependence (a phenomenon in which slower heart rates result in greater APD prolongation), instability, and dispersion of repolarization (an analysis known as TRIaD) appears to be a very powerful analytical tool to predict a drug's risk of inducing arrhythmias.

Changes in the morphology of the T wave

The T wave on the electrocardiogram (ECG) is a marker of ventricular repolarization that represents a multitude of physiological events, including dispersions of repolarization occurring within the thickness of the ventricular walls and between the apex and base of the heart. Drug-induced changes in the morphology of the T wave could also help predict proarrhythmia in the setting of QT prolongation. A revealing clinical study quantitatively analyzed T wave morphology, in addition to QT duration, in 37 patients administered sertindole to explore for drug-induced changes in the T wave that accompany QT prolongation (Nielsen *et al.*, 2009). T wave morphology was assessed by measuring the degree of T wave asymmetry, flatness, and the appearance of notches. Sertindole was shown to induce notable changes in the shape of the T wave; compared to baseline recordings, T waves were significantly more asymmetrical and flat and several patients had notched T waves (Nielsen *et al.*, 2009). Furthermore, the observed changes in T wave morphology were significantly greater than increases in the QT interval. One of the key findings emerging from this study is the fact that in a subset of patients, distinct changes in T wave morphology were recorded despite no QT prolongation.

Changes in T wave morphology have also been identified in patients with congenital long QT syndrome type 2 (LQT 2). As discussed in Chapter 3, the cellular bases for LQT 2 are loss-of-function mutations in the HERG K^+ channel, which is similar in many respects to drug-induced QT prolongation due to HERG blockade;

studies of LQT 2 syndrome may therefore also increase our understanding of drug-induced QT prolongation and proarrhythmia.

An insightful clinical report sought to develop criteria to identify abnormal T wave morphology parameters, in patients with drug-induced QT prolongation, by initially studying ECG parameters in patients with LQT 2 (Graff *et al.*, 2009). Measurements of T wave morphology, similar to those employed in the clinical study of sertindole (T wave asymmetry, flatness, and notching) were conducted in 30 LQT 2 patients and in over 900 healthy subjects to develop a T wave morphology combination score (MCS). Following this initial study, 39 healthy volunteers were administered increasing doses of sotalol over a three-day period and their ECGs were recorded for over 22 hours each day. The MCS was shown to be significantly more sensitive than standard QT measurements in identifying the effects of sotalol on the ECG; even when patients' plasma concentrations of sotalol reached peak values, changes in the QT interval were significantly lower than those of the MCS (Graff *et al.*, 2009).

Measurements of $T_{peak} - T_{end}$

Research that was initially conducted in the isolated ventricular wedge model, simultaneously measuring APs from epicardial, endocardial, and M-cell regions in the left ventricular wall, in addition to a simple form of a single lead ECG, identified that the duration of the T wave corresponded to repolarization times in different regions of the heart (Yan *et al.*, 1998). In particular, measurements of the T wave's duration from its peak to the point at which it returns to baseline (the $T_{peak} - T_{end}$ interval) are considered to be a marker for transmural dispersion of repolarization (TDR) in the ventricular wedge preparation. In ventricular wedge experiments, the peak of the T wave has been shown to correspond to the time at which the epicardium has been fully repolarized and the end of the T wave coincides with complete repolarization of the M-cell layer (Yan *et al.*, 1998). As alterations in the TDR are considered to be an important mechanism underlying ventricular arrhythmias, measurements of the $T_{peak} - T_{end}$ interval on the ECG could potentially be an additional marker of arrhythmia risk in patients. Although no large scale, prospective clinical study has been conducted to assess the power of $T_{peak} - T_{end}$ measurements to predict drug-induced arrhythmias, several reports have provided evidence supporting the utility of this measurement. For example, in one clinical study of patients with drug- or disease-induced QT prolongation, $T_{peak} - T_{end}$ measurements were demonstrated to be strong predictors of arrhythmia risk in patients (Yamaguchi *et al.*, 2003). $T_{peak} - T_{end}$ measurements have also been shown to predict the risk of arrhythmia-induced sudden cardiac death in patients with hypertrophic cardiomyopathy (Shimizu *et al.*, 2002).

Despite these supporting clinical studies, and convincing experimental data using the ventricular wedge model, reports have cast doubt upon the ability of $T_{peak} - T_{end}$ to be a marker of TDR. Using an *in vivo* model, one report concluded that $T_{peak} - T_{end}$ measurements did not represent transmural repolarization gradients but instead reflected total dispersion of repolarization (Opthof *et al.*, 2007). Although $T_{peak} - T_{end}$ measurements do appear to correlate strongly with TDR values in the ventricular wedge model, in the whole heart, where many more cell types and repolarization gradients are present, it is unlikely that $T_{peak} - T_{end}$ measurements reflect only the TDR. Additionally, the optimal methodologies for measuring the $T_{peak} - T_{end}$ interval on the ECG are unclear.

Recent Case Studies of Drug-Induced Proarrhythmia

In the following sections, two recent examples of drug-induced QT prolongation are examined. Both drugs are non-cardiovascular agents and their adverse effects on the heart triggered important changes to their availability in the United States; propoxyphene was withdrawn from the market while a contraindication was added to dolasetron's label. These case studies detail the evidence linking the drugs to cardiac toxicity and describe how the FDA went about determining their safety profiles using preclinical and clinical cardiac safety tests. It is noteworthy that in both of these examples, retrospective clinical safety evaluations were initiated which highlight the fact that, in addition to emerging therapies, current drugs may also be subjected to contemporary cardiac safety testing.

Propoxyphene-Induced Cardiac Toxicity

On November 19th, 2010 the FDA announced that the makers of propoxyphene, an opioid analgesic, had agreed to withdraw the drug from the U.S. market due to the risk of proarrhythmic effects on the heart. Despite the use of propoxyphene since 1957, only recently were its precise adverse effects on the heart documented. New data preceded an FDA re-evaluation of the drug's risk — benefit profile; the FDA concluded that propoxyphene's risk of inducing potentially lethal heart rhythm abnormalities outweighs its therapeutic analgesic effects. The case of propoxyphene-induced cardiac toxicity represents an important example of an older drug, approved long before drug-induced HERG blockade was recognized as a proarrhythmic mechanism of action, being retrospectively subjected to current safety testing procedures.

Clinical and Experimental Studies of Propoxyphene-Induced Cardiac Toxicity

Reports of propoxyphene's adverse effects on the heart, including bradycardia, broadening of the QRS complex, and reduced cardiac contractility, were originally ascribed to cases of overdose with the drug (Strom *et al.*, 1985; Barraclough *et al.*, 1982; Amsterdam *et al.*, 1982). Whereas early reports demonstrated that propoxyphene's neurological adverse effects in cases of drug overdose could be reversed with naloxone administration, cardiac adverse events were on the whole refractory to naloxone treatment. Despite medical interventions to treat propoxyphene's cardiotoxic effects, such as treatment with beta-adrenergic agonists to increase heart rate, the rate of mortality due to cardiac abnormalities was high. One report studying over 200 clinical cases of propoxyphene overdose demonstrated a mortality rate of 8%; cardiovascular causes were implicated in over 75% of these cases (Sloth Madsen *et al.*, 1984). These observations suggested that propoxyphene exerted direct effects on the heart, independent of its analgesic effects.

One of the most revealing studies of propoxyphene-induced cardiac toxicity was a report detailing the case of a female patient admitted to hospital following propoxyphene overdose (Whitcomb *et al.*, 1989). Although the patient's QRS interval was initially within the normal range, significant broadening of the QRS complex was observed in the following four hours despite no further administration of propoxyphene and gastric lavage and administration of activated charcoal (QRS prolongation is illustrated in Figure 8). These delayed effects were considered to have arisen due to propoxyphene's metabolite, norpropoxyphene, which accumulates in cardiac tissue, has a longer half-life, and is approximately two times more potent in depressing cardiac function than propoxyphene (Whitcomb *et al.*, 1989; Ulens *et al.*, 1999). This clinical report also demonstrated that administration of lidocaine, a class 1B antiarrhythmic drug that blocks the Na^+ current, reduced the patient's QRS interval. These clinical observations were corroborated with electrophysiological recordings in isolated rabbit atrial

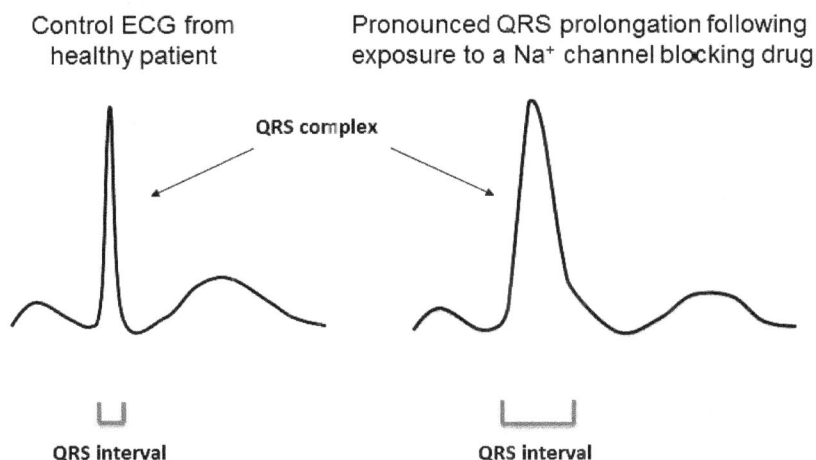

Figure 8: An illustrative example of drug-induced QRS prolongation seen on an ECG recording.

myocytes in which propoxyphene was shown to exert potent blockade of the Na^+ current; this effect of the drug on the Na^+ current was impaired in the presence of lidocaine (Whitcomb *et al.*, 1989).

While propoxyphene's effects on cardiac depolarization and the QRS interval have been described in detail, relatively few reports have studied the drug's effects on cardiac repolarization. Ulens and colleagues' study (1999) of propoxyphene on the HERG K^+ channel was the first report to describe the drug's ability to block this major repolarizing current. In this study, the authors assessed the effects of a range of propoxyphene and norpropoxyphene concentrations on the HERG current; while lower concentrations of the drugs yielded an increase in repolarizing current, much higher concentrations actually reduced the HERG current (Ulens *et al.*, 1999). These results therefore suggest that propoxyphene and norpropoxyphene may exert differential effects on cardiac repolarization across a broad range of concentrations.

A much earlier report assessed the effects of propoxyphene and norpropoxyphene in animal cardiac tissue and in conscious animals (Holland *et al.*, 1979). Using AP recordings from Purkinje fibers, this study demonstrated that both drugs reduced the maximum rate of rise of the AP; this finding suggests a direct effect of the drugs on the cardiac Na^+ channel. Also, at concentrations similar to those used by Ulens and colleagues to induce increases in the HERG current, Holland *et al.* (1979) found that both drugs significantly reduced the APD by approximately 15%. The effects of propoxyphene and its metabolite on a number of ECG parameters were also evaluated in conscious animals. Plasma concentrations of propoxyphene and norpropoxyphene ranging from 1.3 to 10.5 µM produced statistically significant QT prolongation and increases in the QRS interval (Holland *et al.*, 1979). Finally, this study demonstrated the ability of both drugs to accumulate in cardiac tissue.

These experimental and clinical findings clearly indicate that propoxyphene and norpropoxyphene potently block cardiac Na^+ channels, which may lead to QRS prolongation, and exert different effects on the HERG K^+ channel, which may lead to reductions in the AP at lower concentrations, and impaired repolarization and QT prolongation at higher concentrations.

Regulatory Assessment of Propoxyphene's Cardiac Safety Profile

The FDA convened an advisory committee in January 2009 to assess propoxyphene's potential for inducing cardiac adverse events. The advisory committee extensively reviewed results from previously conducted preclinical studies but they concluded that the drug's risk-benefit profile in patients was difficult to determine based on the preclinical studies alone. The advisory committee returned a 14–12 vote against the continued marketing of propoxyphene in the U.S. Additionally, the committee concurred that further information on propoxyphene's cardiac safety profile were needed.

Following the advisory committee meeting, in July 2009 the FDA decided against withdrawing propoxyphene from the U.S. market, presumably until more clinical data on the drug's potential for cardiac adverse effects could be obtained. In Europe, however, the European Medicines Agency recommended that the marketing of propoxyphene should be suspended. The FDA requested that propoxyphene's manufacturer conduct a TQT study which would conclusively determine the drug's proarrhythmic risk. Prior to initiating propoxyphene's TQT study, determination of a supratherapeutic dose of the drug was needed; a preliminary clinical study to assess the effects of ascending doses of propoxyphene was thus conducted. In the FDA's announcement of propoxyphene's withdrawal (FDA, 2010a), the agency described that this supratherapeutic dose determination study was prematurely halted due to safety concerns. In this study, 600 and 900 mg of propoxyphene were associated with QT prolongation of 29.8 and 38.2 ms, respectively; such QT prolongation far exceeds the limits recommended in the ICH E14 guidelines. These prominent clinical findings demonstrated the potentially proarrhythmic effects of propoxyphene, which undoubtedly catalyzed its removal from the U.S. market.

Dolasetron-Induced Cardiac Toxicity

On December 17th, 2010 the FDA announced that the use of IV dolasetron for the management of nausea and vomiting in the setting of cancer chemotherapy was to be contraindicated on the drug's label due to the risk of ventricular arrhythmias. This action was prompted by the findings of a TQT study that the agency had requested which revealed that dolasetron, at both therapeutic and supratherapeutic doses, induced QT prolongation. Similar to the previous examination of propoxyphene's cardiac safety profile, the case of dolasetron also provides an important example of retrospective evaluation of a drug's safety profile despite its long standing clinical use.

Clinical and Experimental Studies of Dolasetron-Induced Cardiac Toxicity

A number of clinical studies of dolasetron have documented its effects on the ECG. One clinical study, a randomized, double-blind study of dolasetron versus ondansetron for the prevention of nausea and vomiting due to chemotherapy, enrolled over 700 hundred patients, 343 of which were administered IV and oral dolasetron. In the dolasetron patient arm, QT prolongation was seen in 41% of patients while QRS prolongation was recorded in 24% of patients (Lofters *et al.*, 1997). The cardiovascular safety profiles of dolasetron and ondansetron have been further assessed in a dedicated clinical study in healthy volunteers administered a range of doses of IV dolasetron (Benedict *et al.*, 1996). Dolasetron induced statistically significant QRS interval prolongation by up to 5.5 ms. Ondansetron failed to evoke similar changes in the QRS interval. However, administration of both dolasetron and ondansetron resulted in significant increases in the QT interval; identical doses of the two drugs prolonged the QT interval by 6.7 and 4.8 ms, respectively (Benedict *et al.*, 1996). Further analyses of the JT interval, an alternative ECG biomarker of repolarization, revealed that only ondansetron significantly prolonged this parameter. Such findings could point to different mechanisms of dolasetron and ondansetron whereby the former predominantly effects cardiac conduction, potentially through the blockade of Na^+ channels, and the latter impairs cardiac repolarization.

Indeed, in keeping with these findings of ondansetron, a cellular study reported that the drug was a potent blocker of the HERG K^+ channel; at a clinically-relevant concentration of 300 nM, ondansetron reduced this ion channel current by 29% (Kuryshev et al., 2000). Despite these effects of dolasetron and ondansetron on ECG biomarkers of depolarization and repolarization, the above clinical study demonstrated that the drug-induced QRS and QT prolongations observed were transient in nature and the duration of these ECG parameters generally returned to baseline values in less than eight hours following drug administration (Benedict et al., 1996).

Several isolated clinical case reports have linked dolasetron's effects on ECG parameters to a range of both atrial and ventricular cardiac arrhythmias, including TdP (Higgins et al., 2005; Turner et al., 2007). In the latter report, two episodes of ventricular fibrillation requiring electrical cardioversion and antiarrhythmic drug therapy were documented shortly following post-surgical administration of dolasetron (Turner et al., 2007). Retrospective assessment of the patient's ECG revealed an episode of TdP prior to VF. Furthermore, a great degree of variability of the QT interval duration (ranging from 460 to 550 ms) was seen before the onset of TdP.

The precise cellular mechanisms underlying these clinical findings were elegantly explored in an *in-vitro* study using mammalian cells expressing the human cardiac Na^+ channel and the HERG and KCNQ1 K^+ channels (Kuryshev et al., 2000). These experiments studied the effects of dolasetron and its major metabolite, MDL 74,156 (MDL). Several clinical studies of dolasetron's pharmacokinetics have shown that the drug is rapidly (within 30 minutes) converted to MDL and that MDL is by far the major pharmacological agent detected in patients (Benedict et al., 1996; Dimmitt et al., 1999). These findings implicate MDL in the cardiac toxicity observed with dolasetron.

Initial experiments revealed that both dolasetron and MDL reduced Na^+ channel currents in a frequency- and concentration-dependent fashion. At a low stimulation frequency even high concentrations (100 µM) of both agents failed to reduce Na^+ channel currents. However, increasing the frequency induced prominent suppression of the Na^+ channel current; 1 μM dolasetron and MDL reduced currents by 21% and 28%, respectively (Kuryshev *et al.*, 2000). Subsequent experiments demonstrated that dolasetron and MDL also reduced the HERG current. Collectively, these findings clearly reveal that both agents have the ability to induce prominent effects on the electrophysiology of the heart which provide a mechanistic basis for the observed QRS and QT prolongation seen in clinical studies.

Regulatory Assessment of Dolasetron's Cardiac Safety Profile

In December 2010 the FDA issued a drug safety communication regarding the potential for dolasteron, in its intravenous form, to induce ECG abnormalities including QT prolongation and TdP when used for the prevention of nausea and vomiting in adult and pediatric patients following chemotherapy (FDA, 2010b). In this safety communication the FDA detailed that this use of dolasetron, in both adult and pediatric patients, was to be contraindicated on the drug's label. However, the use of dolasetron for controlling nausea and vomiting following surgical procedures is still permitted as lower doses of the drug are used in this setting. In keeping with the propoxyphene case study, this safety alert and contraindication for dolasetron were based on new clinical safety findings from a TQT study of dolasetron which revealed that the drug caused QRS and QT prolongation, and thus substantially raised the risk of ventricular arrhythmias such as TdP.

Prior to the FDA's safety alert, dolasetron's cardiac safety profile had been previously noted by the agency and its label did include a warning relating to its potential to induce ECG abnormalities. However, no TQT study of dolasetron had been conducted which precluded in depth characterization of its proarrhymic risk. Accordingly, the FDA recommended that dolasetron's license holder conduct a TQT study using therapeutic and supratherapeutic doses of the drug in adult patients. In this 80 patient, moxifloxacin-controlled study, QT prolongation of 14.1 and 36.6 ms was documented for the therapeutic and supratherapeutic doses of the drug, respectively. Therapeutic and supratherapeutic doses also evoked QRS prolongation in the TQT study. Despite the use of dolasetron in pediatric populations, clinical safety studies in these patients were not conducted; the FDA cited the variability of heart rates in pediatric patients as an important factor precluding the study and interpretation of dolasetron's effects in this patient population (for a further discussion of drug-induced arrhythmias in pediatric patients, please see Chapter 7). For the purposes of determining dolasetron's cardiac safety profile in pediatric patients, simulations of the drug's effects on the pediatric ECG were calculated based on dolasetron's pharmacokinetic properties in these patients; the recommended pediatric dose of dolasetron was calculated to induce QT prolongation of 22.5 ms which is substantially greater than the level of QT prolongation seen in adults. In light of these TQT study findings, IV administration of dolasetron for the management of nausea and vomiting in patients receiving chemotherapy was considered to increase the risk of ECG abnormalities, including arrhythmias.

Summary

Based on recommendations from the ICH guidelines, all new pharmaceuticals undergo preclinical testing to determine their potential effects on cardiac repolarization. Several preclinical cardiac safety systems have been developed, ranging from single cell preparations through to *in vivo* animal models, which provide detailed information of a drug's cardiac safety profile. Generally speaking, preclinical models are positioned to provide different types of cardiac safety information. For example, single cell preparations can be used to determine if a drug blocks a particular ion channel; studies using cardiac tissue or isolated hearts can determine if a drug delays repolarization, alters the heart's electrical heterogeneity, and induces arrhythmias. The TQT study, as described in the ICH E14 guidelines, represented a defining moment in the history of drug safety assessment. Thorough QT studies provide crucial information on the potential of drugs to induce QT prolongation in humans. Early evidence suggests that the predictive power of preclinical and clinical studies could be increased through the use of a number of additional biomarkers, such as repolarization variability and T wave morphology measurements.

References

Amsterdam, E. *et al.* (1982). Depression of myocardial contractile function by propoxyphene and norpropoxyphene. *J Cardiovasc Pharmacol*, **3**, 129–138.

Antzelevith, C. *et al.* (2001). Transmural dispersion of repolarization and the T wave. *Cardiovasc Res*, **50**, 426–431.

Barraclough, C. *et al.* (1982). Failure of naloxone to reverse the cardiotoxicity of distalgesic overdose. *Postgrad Med J*, **58**, 667–668.

Benedict, C. *et al.* (1996). Single-blind study of the effects of intravenous dolasetron mesylate versus ondansetron on electrocardiographic parameters in normal volunteers. *J Cardiovasc Pharmacol*, **28**, 53–59.

Dimmitt, D. *et al.* (1999). Intravenous pharmacokinetics and absolute oral bioavailability of dolasetron in healthy volunteers: part 1. *Biopharm Drug Disp*, **20**, 29–39.

Farkas, A. *et al.* (2008). Importance of vagally mediated bradycardia for the induction of torsade de pointes in an *in vivo* model. *Br J Pharmacol*, **154**, 958–970.

FDA (2010a). Safety Announcement (2010). FDA recommends against the continued use of propoxyphene.

FDA (2010b). Drug Safety Communication: abnormal heart rhythms associated with use of Anzemet (dolasetron mesylate), December 17th, 2010.

Gintant, G. *et al.* (2001). The canine Purkinje fiber: an *in vitro* model system for acquired long QT syndrome and drug-induced arrhythmogenesis. *J Cardiovasc Pharmacol*, **37**, 607–618.

Graff, C. *et al.* (2009). Identifying drug-induced repolarization abnormalities from distinct ECG patterns in congenital long QT syndrome: a study of sotalol effects on T wave morphology. *Drug Safety*, **32**, 599–611.

Higgins, D. *et al.* (2005). Dolasetron and peri-operative cardiac arrhythmia. *Anaesthesia*, **60**, 936–937.

Hinterseer, M. *et al.* (2008). Beat-to-beat variability of QT intervals is increased in patients with drug-induced long QT syndrome: a case control pilot study. *Eur Heart J.* **29**, 185–190.

Holland, D. *et al.* (1979). Electrophysiologic properties of propoxyphene and norpropoxyphene in canine cardiac conducting tissues *in vitro* and *in vivo. Toxicol Appl Pharmacol*, **47**, 123–133.

Hondeghem, L. *et al.* (2001). Instability and triangulation of the action potential predict serious proarrhythmia, but action potential duration prolongation is antiarrhythmic. *Circulation*, **103**, 2004–2013.

ICH (2005a). The non-clinical evaluation of the potential for delayed ventricular repolarization (QT interval prolongation) by human pharmaceuticals S7B. International Conference on Harmonization of Technical Requirements for Registration of Pharmaceuticals for Human Use. www.ich.org/fileadmin/Public_Web_Site/ICH_Products/Guidelines/Safey/ S7B/Step4/S7B_Guideline.pdf (accessed March 4th, 2011).

ICH (2005b). The Clinical Evaluation of QT/QTc Interval Prolongation and Proarrhythmic Potential for Non-Antiarrhythmic Drugs E14. International Conference on Harmonization. www.ich.org/fileadmin/ Public_Web_Site/ICH_Products/Guidelines/Efficacy/E14/Step4/ E14_Guideline.pdf (accessed March 4th, 2011).

Kääb, S. *et al.* (2003). Sotalol testing unmasks altered repolarization in patients with suspected acquired long-QT-syndrome — a case-control pilot study using i.v. sotalol. *Eur Heart J*, **24**, 649–657.

Killeen, M. *et al.* (2007). Arrhythmogenic mechanisms in the isolated perfused hypokalemic murine heart. *Acta Physiol*, **189**, 33–46.

Kuryshev, Y. *et al.* (2000). Interactions of the 5-hydroxytryptamine 3 antagonist class of antiemetic drugs with human cardiac ion channels. *J Pharm Exp Ther*, **295**, 614–620.

Lofters, W. *et al.* (1997). Phase III double-blind comparison of dolasetron mesylate and ondansetron and an evaluation of the additive role of dexamethasone in the prevention of acute and delayed nausea and vomiting due to moderately emetogenic chemotherapy. *J Clin Oncol*, **15**, 2966–2967.

Lu, H. *et al.* (2001). Species plays an important role in drug-induced prolongation of action potential duration and early afterdepolarizations in isolated Purkinje fibers. *J Cardiovasc Electrophysiol*, **12**, 93–102.

Mantravadi, R. *et al.* (2007). Autonomic nerve stimulation reverses ventricular repolarization sequence in rabbit hearts. *Circ Res*, **100**, 72–80.

Michael, G. *et al.* (2008). Adrenaline reveals the torsadogenic effect of combined blockade of potassium channels in anaesthetized guinea pigs. *Br J Pharmacol*, **154**, 1414–1426.

Milberg, P. *et al.* (2002). Divergent proarrhythmic potential of macrolide antibiotics despite similar QT prolongation: fast phase 3 repolarization prevents early afterdepolarizations and torsade de pointes. *J Pharmacol Exp Ther*, **303**, 218–225.

Nielsen, J. *et al.* (2009). Sertindole causes distinct electrocardiographic T wave morphology changes. *Eur Neuropsychopharmacol*, **19**, 702–707.

Opthof, T. *et al.* (2007). Dispersion of repolarization in canine ventricle and the electrocardiographic T wave: Tp-e interval does not reflect transmural dispersion. *Heart Rhythm*, **4**, 341–348.

Shimizu, M. *et al.* (2002). T-peak to T-end interval may be a better predictor of high-risk patients with hypertrophic cardiomyopathy associated with a cardiac troponin I mutation than QT dispersion. *Clin Cardiol*, **25**, 335–339.

Sloth Madsen, P. *et al.* (1984). Acute propoxyphene self-poisoning in 222 consective patients. *Acta Anaesthesiol Scand*, **28**, 661–665.

Strom, J. *et al.* (1985). The effects of naloxone on central hemodynamics and myocardial metabolism in experimental propoxyphene-induced circulatory shock. *Acta Anaesthesiol Scand*, **29**, 693–697.

Sugiyama, S. *et al.* (2008). Sensitive and reliable proarrhythmia *in vivo* animal models for predicting drug-induced torsades de pointes in patients with remodelled hearts. *B J Pharmacol*, **154**, 1528–1537.

Thomsen, M. *et al.* (2006). Beat-to-beat variability of repolarization determines proarrhythmic outcome in dogs susceptible to drug-induced torsades de pointes. *J Am Col Cardiol*, **48**, 1268–1276.

Turner, S. *et al.* (2007). Dolasetron-induced torsades de pointes. *J Clin Anesth*, **19**, 622–625.

Ulens, C. *et al.* (1999). Norpropoxyphene-induced cardiotoxicity is associated with changes in ion-selectivity and gating of HERG currents. *Cardiovasc Res*, **44**, 568–578.

Varró, A. *et al.* (2001). Electrophysiological effects of Dronedarone (SR 33589), a non-iodinated amiodarone derivative in the canine heart: comparison with amiodarone. *Br J Pharmacol*, **133**, 625–634.

Whitcomb, D. *et al.* (1989). Marked QRS complex abnormalities and sodium channel blockade by propoxyphene reversed with lidocaine. *J Clin Invest*, **84**, 1629–1636.

Yamaguchi, M. *et al.* (2003). T wave peak-to-end interval and QT dispersion in acquired long QT syndrome: a new index for arrhythmogenicity. *Clin Sci (Lond)*, **105**, 671-676.

Yamamoto, K. *et al.* (2001). Acute canine model for drug-induced Torsades de Pointes in drug safety evaluation-influences of anesthesia and validation with quinidine and astemizole. *Toxicol Sci*, **60**,165–176.

Yan, G. *et al.* (1998). Cellular basis for the normal T wave and the electrocardiographic manifestations of the long-QT syndrome. *Circulation*, **98**, 1928–1936.

CHAPTER 7

Pediatric Cardiac Safety

Introduction

As discussed in the previous chapters, the ability of drugs to induce cardiac arrhythmias and sudden death has been one of the leading causes behind a number of high profile drug withdrawals, spanning multiple indications, in the last decade. A number of reports, dating back to 1996, have documented cases of children presenting with a range of cardiovascular complications due to drugs that impair repolarization through HERG blockade. The physiology and pharmacology of the mammalian heart changes significantly throughout development. For example, it is well known that the human heart undergoes significant electrophysiological changes as it develops; these electrical changes take place at the ion channel level. Despite the in-depth preclinical assessment of new drugs during the drug development process, cardiac safety studies are predominantly performed in adult tissue and experimental models. Evidence suggests that pediatric patients are susceptible to a wide array of drug-induced proarrhythmic effects, that in some cases contrast sharply with those seen in adults, and that a patient's age may dictate the risk of cardiac toxicity. The aims of this chapter are to review previous preclinical studies and clinical case reports of drug-induced pediatric cardiac toxicity and to explore the potential mechanisms underlying these events.

Cisapride-Induced Pediatric Cardiac Toxicity

One of the first reports of cisapride-induced QT prolongation in a pediatric patient was described by Lewin and colleagues in 1996 in which a two-month-old patient receiving cisapride presented with a QT interval of 510 ms in addition to 2:1 AV block and a variable T wave morphology (Lewin *et al.*, 1996). Since this initial description several reports have described cisapride-induced delays in repolarization in cohorts of pediatric patients. Pediatric drug-induced QT prolongation, in the absence of ventricular arrhythmias, has also been reported with doxapram, droperidol, and atypical antopsychotic therapy (for a succinct review of drugs associated with QT prolongation in pediatric patients see Buck, 2005).

Several reports studying the effects of cisapride therapy in pediatric patients of different ages have also revealed that the drug's ability to induct QT prolongation is sharply correlated with a patient's age. One of the most enlightening descriptions of these age-dependent effects of cisapride was a study by Dubin and colleagues in 2001. In their report, Dubin *et al.* (2001) measured the QT interval and JT interval before and after cisapride administration in 25 pediatric patients with gestational ages ranging from 27–34 weeks (for the purposes of their analyses, two patient groups were studied — patients ≤ 31 weeks of age and those >31 weeks of age). Measuring the JT interval has been proposed to offer several advantages over QT interval measurements; the QT interval captures both ventricular depolarization and repolarization, thus conduction abnormalities could interfere with the interpretation of the QT interval when it is being used as a marker of repolarization.

In the Dubin study, prior to drug administration QT and JT intervals were not significantly different in the two patient groups (the mean QT intervals were 410 and 400 ms and the mean JT intervals were 340 and 330 ms in the ≤31-week and >31-week patients, respectively). However, following cisapride therapy in the ≤31-week patient group, the QT interval significantly increased to 440 ms ($P \le 0.05$); although QT prolongation was also seen in the >31-week study group, the increase was not statistically significant from baseline recordings. Cisapride also induced a statistically significant increase in the JT interval to 370 ms in the ≤31-week patient group, effects not seen in the older patients. Dubin and colleagues (2001) also assessed the ability of cisapride to induce pathological QT and JT prolongation in pediatric patients; in their study, a QT interval ≥450 ms and a JT interval ≥360 ms were considered to be pathological. QT interval prolongation ≥450 ms was seen in 32% patients while pathological JT prolongation was documented in 40% patients and 90% of these patients were ≤31 weeks of age. These results demonstrate a striking age-related effect of cisapride in which younger patients were more susceptible to pathological drug-induced delays in repolarization. Despite these notable increases in the QT interval no arrhythmias were reported in this clinical study. This observation could have resulted from either the low proarrhythmic liability of QT prolonging drugs in young patients or the degree of medical intervention used in the study. For example, cisapride therapy could have been discontinued in patients with a QT interval ≥450 ms to reduce the risk of cardiac adverse events.

These findings by Dubin and colleagues echo those of an earlier study by Bernardini *et al.* (1997). This investigation was a survey of infants that had been administered cisapride between 1995 and 1996, with ECGs conducted before and approximately two days after the initiation of drug therapy; in keeping with the Dubin report, Bernardini and colleagues (1997) defined QT intervals ≥450 ms as pathological. The effects of cisapride on the QT interval were assessed in 49 patients with a mean gestational age of 34.6 weeks; cisapride induced a statistically significant increase in the QT interval from mean values of 395 ms to 418 ms (P = 0.0001). Moreover, pathological QT prolongation was seen in 14% of patients, 85% of which were ≤33 weeks of age, thus also demonstrating a close correlation between age and the risk of severe drug-induced QT prolongation. Importantly, Bernardini *et al.* (1997) also reported that the QT prolongation observed with cisapride was not associated with ventricular arrhythmias.

A third study of cisapride-induced QT prolongation in pediatric patients was amongst the first to report drug-induced TdP in this patient population (Hill *et al.*, 1998). In their study, Hill and colleagues (1998) monitored the effects of cisapride on the QT interval in 35 patients of a much larger age range compared to the two studies described above. QT and JT intervals in addition to other potential proarrhythmia biomarkers, such as QT dispersion and JT dispersion, were measured. Hill *et al.* (1998) demonstrated that cisapride therapy did not result in a statistically significant increase in mean QT prolongation (420 vs. 430 ms in the control and drug-treated groups, respectively); however, QT prolongation ≥ 450 ms was seen in 13% patients and JT interval prolongation ≥ 360 ms was observed in 46% of patients. Dispersion in the QT or JT interval greater than 70 ms was only seen in three patients (9%), which could imply that cisapride has a relatively limited capacity for inducing prominent repolarization heterogeneity in pediatric patients. Nevertheless, one of the more intriguing findings from this study was the documented incidence of TdP in two patients presenting with a QT ≥ 450 ms; however, in contrast to the patients studied in the Dubin and Bernardini reports, these two patients were considerably older (12 and 14 years of age) and they were receiving concomitant macrolide antibacterial therapy, which is known to impair the metabolism of other drugs through inhibition of the hepatic CYP-450 enzymes (cisapride, for example, is metabolized by the CYP-450 enzyme family). With these considerations in mind, these two cases of cisapride-induced TdP closely correlate with notable case reports of drug-induced TdP seen in adult patients. However, extrapolation of these clinical findings to the broader, younger pediatric patient population is limited due to the older age of these patients and their use of concomitant drugs.

Potential Mechanisms Underlying Cisapride-Induced Cardiac Toxicity in Pediatric Patients

Now that we have examined in close detail these three reports of cisapride-induced QT prolongation in pediatric patients it is important to consider some of the underlying mechanisms that could be responsible for these observations, in which greater degrees of QT prolongation are seen in younger patients. Due to our knowledge of cisapride's effects in adults, two principal, and not necessarily independent, pathophysiological mechanisms could explain the drug's effects in pediatric patients: (1) a reduced capacity for cisapride metabolism and (2) lower levels of repolarization capacity in the pediatric heart compared to the adult heart.

Cisapride is metabolized by subtype 3A4 of the CYP-450 hepatic enzyme family; the function of this metabolic enzyme could be suboptimal in younger patients, which could result in greater plasma levels of cisapride and therefore an increased risk of cardiac toxicity. In the following sections, the potential direct effects of cisapride on the heart are discussed.

The proarrhythmic effects of drugs in the developing heart

The physiology of the heart changes significantly during development. The heart's electrophysiological profile during development appears to be in a constant state of flux at the cellular level, with a number of ionic currents being up- and down-regulated. Current adult-based experimental models that are routinely used in preclinical cardiac safety studies might not be able to account for these significant developmental changes in cardiac electrophysiology.

An important study identified the electrophysiological and pharmacological differences between neonatal, young and adult animal hearts and determined the pathological consequences of QT prolongation during development (Obreztchikova *et al.*, 2003). The effects of dofetilide were examined in animal prepations of varying age; neonatal (approximately eight days), young (approximately 90 days) and adult (three to five years) canine preparations were used. *In vivo* ECG recordings revealed that dofetilide consistently induced prominent QT prolongation across all ages studied, the magnitude of which was similar in neonatal, young, and adult preparations. Based on these findings alone, one could assume that the cardiac electrophysiological profiles across all three age groups would be similar;

however, subsequent cellular recordings taken from epicardial ventricular myocytes revealed vastly different findings between neonatal and adult animals that have implications for drug safety testing.

In the Obreztchikova study (2003), action potentials (APs) recorded from ventricular myocytes in the absence of any drugs had a triangular morphology that lacked the characteristic Phase 1 that is due to the effects of the I_{to} current. In neonatal hearts, while dofetilide induced AP duration (APD) prolongation, azimilide (a known blocker of the KCNQ1 K$^+$ channel) failed to evoke further changes in APD, suggesting the absence of the KCNQ1 K$^+$ current at this developmental stage. On the other hand, APs recorded from adult animals were sensitive to dofetilide and azimilide and both drugs induced APD prolongation, indicating the presence of functional HERG and KCNQ1 K$^+$ channels (Obreztchikova *et al.*, 2003). In further experiments the transmural dispersion of repolarization (TDR) was measured in neonatal, young, and adult cardiac tissue by recording APs from endocardial, M-cell, and epicardial regions; at baseline, while TDR was found to be minimal in neonatal hearts, it steadily increased with age. Furthermore, the effects of dofetilide on the TDR were strongly dependent on age; the smallest increase in TDR was shown to occur in neonatal preparations and the greatest increase was found in adult cardiac tissue (Obreztchikova *et al.*, 2003).

In further experiments Obreztchikova and colleagues (2003) studied the arrhythmogenic consequences of dofetilide administration in neonatal, young, and adult animals by recording the incidence of triggered activity and TdP arrhythmias. Intriguingly, despite prominent QT prolongation in neonates administered dofetilide, triggered activity and ventricular arrhythmias were not observed. In young animals, triggered activity and TdP were recorded in 59% and 29% of preparations, respectively. In adults, the incidence of these arrhythmic events was lower — triggered activity and TdP were detected in only 20% of preparations (Obreztchikova *et al.*, 2003). Collectively, the findings from this insightful study suggest that neonates have a very low risk of drug-induced ventricular arrhythmias despite the ability of drugs to impair repolarization and induce significant QT prolongation. The study also indicates that following the neonatal stage, there is a period of time in which the risk of TdP transiently increases prior to the adult stage. Such findings may result from the development of key Ca^{2+} handling proteins in the heart, such as the maturation of the sarcoplasmic reticulum or the regulation of L-type Ca^{2+} channels, which could lead to abnormalities in Ca^{2+} homeostasis and a high rate of EADs which could trigger TdP arrhythmias. Additionally, these developmental changes in Ca^{2+} handling could coincide with the appearance of a small, but sufficient TDR seen in the young animals.

These observations with dofetilide in animals of varying age, coupled with clinical reports of cisapride, in which the drug induced a greater magnitude of QT prolongation in younger patients, clearly suggest that developmental changes in repolarizing K^+ channels may play an important role in mediating the effects of drug-induced HERG blockade in pediatric patients. An insightful study by Grandy and colleagues (2007) studied changes in the APD and related these findings to levels of individual K^+ channels in the mouse heart. Although important species-related differences in cardiac electrophysiology must be acknowledged, this report nevertheless provides a useful framework for understanding the effects of impaired repolarization in the developing heart. Briefly, APs and K^+ currents were recorded from ventricular myocytes from mice of varying ages (adult animals and those at ages of one, seven and 20 days were assessed). Grandy *et al.* (2007) demonstrated that the ventricular AP changes significantly throughout development. Waveforms recorded from one-day-old myocytes had a distinct plateau that was not seen in APs recorded from myocytes from older animals. Action potential durations also varied with development; the APD significantly decreased with age. Measurements of K^+ currents were also significantly different in the four age populations with levels of I_{to} and I_{K1} being significantly greater in older animal hearts. Similar age-related changes in ventricular repolarization have also been seen in the rabbit (Valverde *et al.*, 2003). Collectively, these studies suggest that the density of ventricular repolarizing K^+ currents increases with age in the developing

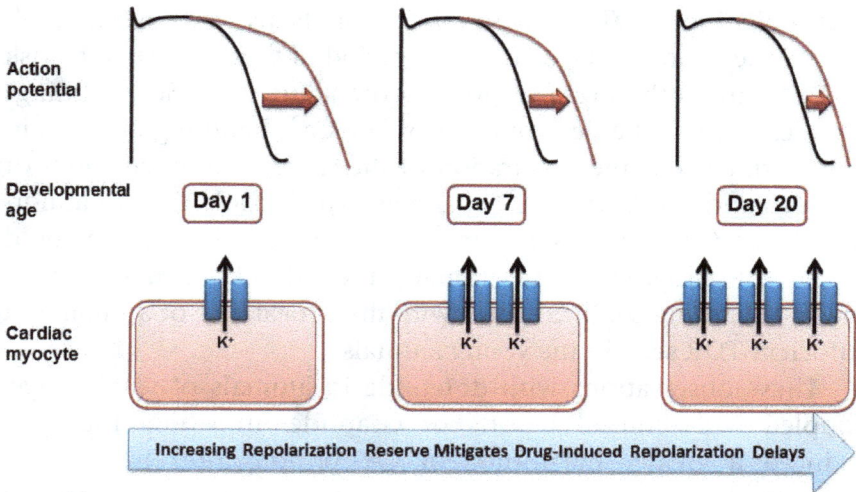

Figure 1:   The upregulation of repolarizing K$^+$ currents during cardiac development and how this may influence the degree of drug-induced action potential duration prolongation.

mammalian heart which results in a corresponding decrease in APD. With these findings in mind, drugs that decrease the level of a single repolarizing K$^+$ current, such as the HERG channel-mediated I_{Kr} K$^+$ current, would be expected to have a greater effect in younger versus older hearts and cause greater degrees of QT prolongation with decreasing age. The upregulation of repolarizing K$^+$ currents with age, and the potential effects of drug-induced HERG blockade on the cardiac APD, are illustrated in Figure 1.

Drug-Induced Cardiac Toxicity in the Embryonic Heart

Studies have revealed that HERG blocking drugs, such as erythromycin, can induce substantial toxicological defects in the developing embryo. Between five and nine weeks of pregnancy, before the embryonic heart is innervated, the heart is susceptible to developing a range of drug-induced congenital defects. Researchers have proposed that low concentrations of medications that pose no risk to the mother, are prone to cause potent HERG K$^+$ channel blockade in the embryonic heart and lead to delays in repolarization and the development of bradycardia. Embryonic bradyarrhythmias cause disruptions in blood flow and alterations in blood pressure which could be responsible for congenital cardiovascular defects. A number of studies have also proposed that drug-induced bradycardia in the embryo may result in hypoxia, the generation of reactive oxygen species, vascular disruption, hemorrhage, and a range of embryonic malformations such as growth retardation, orofacial defects and heart vessel defects (Azarbayjani *et al.*, 2002; Danielsson *et al.*, 2001; Kallen *et al.*, 2005).

One of the most insightful studies linking repolarization-related embryonic cardiac toxicity to developmental defects investigated the electrophysiological mechanisms underlying the ability of commonly used antiepileptic medications to induce teratogenic effects (Azarbayjani *et al.*, 2002). Trimethadione has been previously associated with a high rate of cardiac defects. Azarbayjani and colleagues (2002) explored for the potential effects of trimethadione, and its metabolite dimethadione, on the embryonic heart. Using a series of *in vivo* and cellular experiments, the researchers demonstrated that dimethadione administration induced embryonic bradycardia; heart rates were reduced by 30% in embryos studied at gestational day (GD) 9 and these bradycardiac effects of the drug persisted for up to 48 hours in which heart rates were reduced by 45% (Azarbayjani *et al.*, 2002). The authors reported that arrhythmias were seen in 57% of embryos 48 hours after administration of dimethadione; however, a precise description of these arrhythmias was not reported. This study also demonstrated the transient nature of dimethadione-induced embryonic cardiotoxicity. The developing heart was susceptible to drug-induced bradycardia at GD 9 through to GD 12; beyond this period, at GD 14 through to GD 16, high concentrations of dimethadione failed to evoke changes to the heart rates of embryos. Subsequent experiments also revealed that dimethadione induced blockade of the HERG K^+ channel (Azarbayjani *et al.*, 2002). The authors of this study also assessed dimethadione's teratogenic effects; dimethadione treatment was associated with an increased rate of fetal mortality, reduced fetal weight, and a 40% incidence of cleft palate (Azarbayjani *et al.*, 2002). While this study did not determine a precise link between the dimethadione-induced bradycardia and teratogenic effects seen with the drug, a speculative pathway was proposed. The ability of dimethadione to induce birth defects, such as cleft palate, was attributed to the drug's disruption of the embryonic cardiac rhythm in which HERG blockade induced episodes of bradycardia, arrhythmia, and asystole which led to disruptions in blood flow and hypoxia during a critical stage of embryonic development. Upon resumption of a normal cardiac rhythm, either due to spontaneous termination of an arrhythmia or the reduced ability of dimethadione to induce bradycardia during later stages of development, reperfusion and the generation of reactive oxygen species could exert adverse effects on the heart resulting in tissue necrosis and the development of malformations. Intriguingly almokalant, a potent HERG K^+ channel blocking drug, has also been shown to induce notable reductions in the heart rates of embryonic rats and increase the rate of fetal mortality (Abrahamsson *et al.*, 1994). With these studies in mind, the cardiotoxic effects of drugs have the potential to induce wide ranging adverse events in the developing embryo. When immature hearts are exposed to HERG blocking drugs, reductions in heart rate and the development of bradyarrhythmias, such as AV block, appear to be common (the possible mechanisms underlying drug-induced AV block in the embryonic heart are depicted in Figure 2). In the embryonic heart, drug-induced delays in repolarization could prove to be particularly harmful by inducing hypoxia and subsequently triggering a range of severe developmental defects, as seen in the animal studies.

Summary

As the mammalian heart matures to its adult state its electrophysiological profile profoundly changes; the level of repolarizing K^+ channels, for example, appears to increase with age. The dynamic nature of the developing heart appears to shape the proarrhythmic potential of a range of drugs that delay repolarization. As seen in animal studies, the responses to drug-induced impaired repolarization appear to be largely

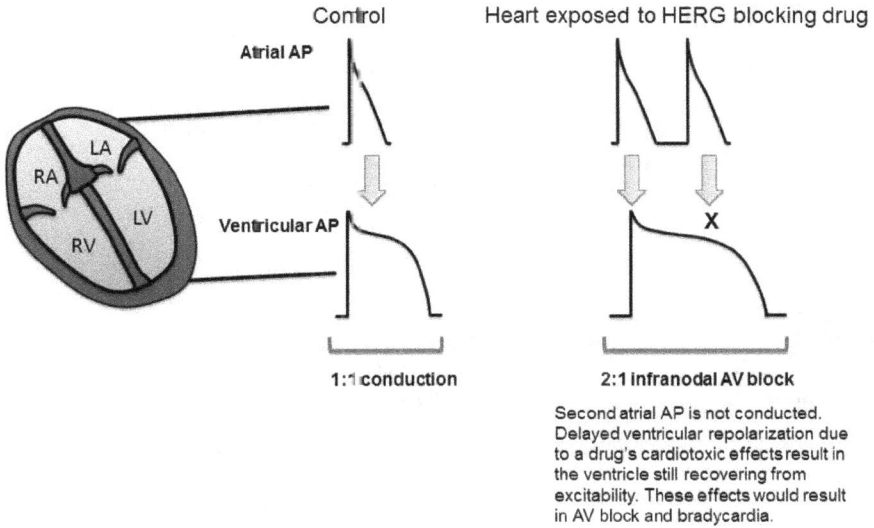

Figure 2:   Potential mechanisms underlying embryonic drug-induced bradycardia.

dictated by the age of the heart; despite significant QT prolongation in neonatal animal hearts, for example, the rates of EADs and arrhythmias were low. In slighter older animals, however, a high rate of EADs led to more frequent episodes of TdP (Obreztchikova *et al.*, 2003). These preclinical findings are, in part, supported by clinical case studies; although drug-induced QT prolongation has been commonly reported in pediatric patients, only a handful of drug-induced TdP cases have been documented. However, there is no evidence suggesting a transient increase in proarrhythmia risk in pediatric patients, as reported in preclinical studies (the correlation between results from the Obreztchikova preclinical study and clinical reports are illustrated in Figure 3). Additionally, drug-induced delays in repolarization can exert notable disturbances in the cardiac rhythm of embryonic hearts, particularly bradycardia and asystole, which induce systemic developmental defects. The evolution of the mammalian heart's susceptibility to drug-induced arrhythmias, and the types of arrhythmias most commonly reported at different ages is depicted in Figure 4. Clearly, further research into the mechanisms, incidence, and consequences of pediatric drug-induced QT prolongation and proarrhythmia is warranted.

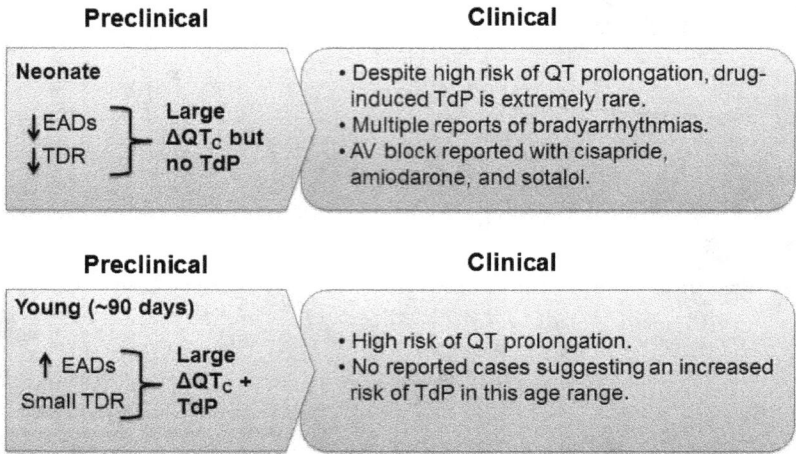

Figure 3: The correlation between preclinical and clinical reports of pediatric cardiac toxicity.

Stage of development →

	Embryonic	Neonatal	Juvenile	Adult
TDR	–	Low	Med	High
EAD risk	–	Low	High?	Low
VT risk	–	Low	Med-High	Low-Med
Arrhythmia	Bradycardia/ asystole	Bradycardia/ AV block	VT/TdP	VT/TdP

Figure 4: The theoretical evolution of a drug's proarrhythmic effects during cardiac development.

References

Abrahamsson, C. *et al*. (1994). Induction of rhythm abnormalities in the fetal rat heart. A tentative mechanism for the embryotoxic effect of the class III antiarrhythmic agent almokalant. *Cardiovasc Res*, **28**, 337–344.

Azarbayjani, F. *et al.* (2002). Embryonic arrhythmia by inhibition of HERG channels: a common hypoxia-related teratogenic mechanism for antiepileptic drugs? *Epilepsia*, 43, 457–468.

Bernardini, S. *et al.* (1997). Effects of cisapride on QTc interval in neonates. *Arch Dis Child Fetal Neonatal Ed*, **77**, F241–F243.

Buck, M. (2005). Drug-induced QT prolongation: examples from the pediatric literature. *Ped Pharmacother*, **11**(10).

Danielsson, B. *et al.* (2001). Class III antiarrhythmics and phenytoin: teratogenicity due to embryonic cardiac dysrhythmia and reoxygenation damage. *Curr Pharm Des*, **7**. 787–802.

Dubin, A. *et al.* (2001). Cisapride associated with QTc prolongation in very low birth weight preterm infants. *Pediatrics*, **107**, 1313–1316.

Grandy, S. *et al.* (2007). Postnatal development has a marked effect on ventricular repolarization in mice. *Am J Physiol Heart Circ Physiol*, **293**, H2168–H2177.

Hill, S. *et al.* (1998). Proarrhythmia associated with cisapride in children. *Pediatrics*, **101**, 1053–1056.

Kallen, B. *et al.* (2005). Is erythromycin therapy teratogenic in humans? *Reprod Toxicol*, **20**, 209–214.

Lewin, M. *et al.* (1996). Cisapride-induced long QT interval. *J Pediatr*, **128**, 279–281.

Obreztchikova, M. *et al.* (2003) Developmental changes in IKr and IKs contribute to age-related expression of dofetilide effects on repolarization and proarrhythmia. *Cardiovasc Res*, **59**, 339–350.

Valverde, S. *et al.* (2003). Developmental changes of cardiac repolarization in rabbits: implications for the role of sex hormones. *Cardiovasc Res*, **57**, 625–631.

CHAPTER 8

Drug-Induced Atrial Fibrillation

Introduction

Based on the mechanisms underlying drug-induced ventricular arrhythmias, where cardioactive drugs alter the function of ion channels, the ability of drugs to exert similarly proarrhythmic effects on the atria remains a distinct possibility. However, relatively little information exists on the incidence and pathological consequences of drug-induced atrial arrhythmias. The vast majority of published studies on this area of cardiac safety are predominantly limited to meta analyses, clinical studies that were not primarily designed to measure cardiac arrhythmias, and isolated clinical case reports. Additionally, in many of these studies, the proarrhythmic mechanisms of drugs linked to atrial fibrillation (AF) were not elucidated. This chapter will provide an overview of drug-induced AF by examining several agents that have been implicated in this common heart rhythm abnormality. The implications of drug-induced AF are also discussed as is the potential for routinely evaluating drugs in safety studies to determine their potential to induce AF.

Atrial Fibrillation

Atrial fibrillation is the most common cardiac arrhythmia encountered in clinical practice and it is an important cause of morbidity and mortality; AF is associated with a five-fold increased risk of thromboembolic stroke compared to patients free from AF

(Camm *et al.*, 2010). The prevalence of AF is sharply correlated with age; AF has previously been estimated to affect 0.5% of the population aged between 40 and 50 years and 5%–15% of the population aged 80 years and over (Camm *et al.*, 2010). Drug treatment strategies for AF are dependent on a range of different factors including existing cardiovascular comorbidities, the severity of the symptoms associated with the arrhythmia, and the specific subtype of AF that the patient presents with. Alongside stroke prevention therapies, through the use of antiplatelet or anticoagulant drugs, current medical practice for managing AF generally falls into two categories — rhythm control or rate control. Highly symptomatic patients with paroxysmal or persistent AF are optimal candidates for rhythm control treatments in which the primary aim is to restore the heart's normal sinus rhythm. In these patients, recent onset AF that fails to self terminate is managed through the use of cardioversion, either electrical or chemical (using antiarrhythmic drugs), and the subsequent use of prophylactic antiarrhythmic drugs to prevent the recurrence of the arrhythmia. Attempts at restoring normal sinus rhythm in patients presenting with long lasting episodes of AF, in addition to other risk factors for AF including age and heart failure, are often not as effective. In these cases, ventricular rate control treatment strategies are often adopted whereby drugs are administered to control the ventricular rate and the AF is allowed to continue. It is not the intention of this section to describe the detailed treatment algorithms of AF; this text represents merely a summary of some of the broader principles of AF management. For thorough descriptions of AF treatment protocols, the reader is encouraged to consult national AF treatment guidelines such as those published by the European Society of Cardiology or the American Heart Association.

Bisphosphonate-Induced Atrial Fibrillation

One of the first reports to initially propose a potential link between the use of bisphosphonates and the development of atrial arrhythmias was a 2007 study of zolendronic acid for the treatment of post-menopausal osteoporosis in 3,889 patients (Black *et al.*, 2007). In this study, 50 patients administered zolendronic acid went on to develop a serious episode of AF compared to 20 patients receiving a placebo, a statistically significant increased risk (P < 0.001) (Black *et al.*, 2007). However, when a small cohort of patients in this study underwent ECG testing, no significant difference in the prevalence of AF was found between the drug-treated and placebo patient groups (2.1% patients in the zolendronic acid group compared to 2.8% patients in the trial's placebo arm) (Black *et al.*, 2007).

A subsequent retrospective study of patients from the Fracture Intervention Trial, a study of oral alendronate in 6,459 post-menopausal women with low bone mass, also revealed a raised risk of developing AF in patients treated with bisphosphontes (Cummings *et al.*, 2007). In this analysis, Cummings and colleagues (2007) reported 47 serious episodes of AF in patients administered alendronate compared to 31 placebo-treated patients (1.5% and 1% incidence of AF, respectively), which approached statistical significance (P = 0.07). Collectively, these findings suggest that bisphosphonate treatment could increase the risk of developing symptomatic episodes of AF that may require hospitalization, possible electrical or chemical cardioversion, and the initiation of anticoagulant therapy to reduce a patient's stroke risk. Since the publication of these clinical reports, a number of other studies have either confirmed these findings, by demonstrating a close causal relationship between bisphosphonate use and AF, or have proposed that drugs belonging to this class pose no risk of AF. Additionally, the potential mechanisms underlying the development of atrial arrhythmias with this drug class remain unclear.

In 2010, a report demonstrated a close correlation between intravenous bisphosphonate use in cancer patients and AF, supraventricular tachycardia (SVT), and stroke (Wilkinson *et al.*, 2010). This study harnessed information contained within the Surveillance, Epidemiology, and End Results Medicare database to retrospectively assess the incidence of these events in 6,857 cancer patients treated with bisphosphonates between 1995 and 2003. Importantly, cancer patients could have a higher risk of cardiac toxicity with these drugs due to the fact that they are typically exposed to high doses of bisphosphonates (cancer patients may receive considerably higher doses of bisphosphonates compared to patients with osteoporosis) and through the use of adjunct chemotherapeutic drugs, such as anthracyclines, which have been previously shown to exert toxic effects on the heart.

In their study, Wilkinson and colleagues (2010) demonstrated that after three years since the initiation of bisphosphonate therapy, AF had been documented in 18% of cancer patients compared to 12.7% of patients not receiving the drugs, these findings translated to an absolute risk difference of 5% — this risk difference was increased to 8% at six years (Wilkinson *et al.*, 2010). Some of the most important findings to emerge from this study concerned the documented incidence of stroke among cancer patients administered bisphosphonates compared to matched non-users of these drugs. The rate of hospitalization due to stroke was 5.5% in the bisphosphonate group compared to 4.1% in the study's control group at three years, an absolute risk of 1.5% which increased to 4% at six years (Wilkinson *et al.*, 2010). In terms of other atrial arrhythmias, the authors reported that after three years the rate of SVT was 28% and 20.4% in bisphosphonate users and control patients, respectively. Overall, use of bisphosphonates in cancer patients in this study was associated with a 30% increased risk of developing AF or suffering from a stroke (Wilkinson *et al.*, 2010).

Despite these convincing findings linking bisphosphonates to the development of AF and stroke, it is important to acknowledge that a number of other studies investigating bisphosphonate-induced cardiac toxicity have reported that these drugs do not raise the risk of developing AF (for a succinct review of the clinical evidence linking bisphosphonates to atrial fibrillation, see Gralow *et al.*, 2010). Furthermore, following an FDA request for placebo-controlled, clinical trial data alongside post-marketing surveillance data for approved bisphosphonate drugs, the agency concluded that there was no prominent link between AF and the use of bisphosphonate drugs. Additionally, another large clinical study failed to find an increased risk of AF in bisphosphonate-treated patients (Arslan *et al.*, 2011).

With such conflicting evidence, what could explain the reports of bisphosphonate-induced AF in cancer patients, and the lack of these findings in other clinical studies? Firstly, all of the above clinical studies were not prospective, dedicated cardiac safety studies of bisphosphonates; it is also unclear how atrial arrhythmias were recorded in these prior clinical/epidemiological studies. For example, although a 12-lead ECG study of 559 patients in the original study linking zolendronic acid to AF (Black *et al.*, 2007) failed to report a higher incidence of the arrhythmia in the patients assigned to the drug, it certainly remains possible that the (presumably) relatively brief monitoring periods failed to correspond to the precise time in which patients were in AF. If the study had incorporated more frequent ECG monitoring in a larger sample of patients, atrial arrhythmias may well have been documented. Finally, it is uncertain how the episodes of AF were graded in terms of severity in the study by Black and colleagues (2007). Furthermore, of the patients developing severe AF, it is unclear what drugs were used to manage these events; did any of the AF episodes spontaneously convert back to a normal sinus rhythm or were electrical or chemical cardioversion procedures used? These questions can only be answered through large-scale prospective clinical trials dedicated to bisphosphonate cardiac safety that incorporate frequent ECG monitoring of patients.

Although the precise cardiotoxic mechanisms that could explain the raised risk of developing AF with bisphosphonate therapy remain unclear, a number of potential adverse effects of these drugs on the atria have been proposed (Pazianas *et al.*, 2010). One insightful study provided direct evidence that alendronate treatment, both acute and long-term, led to the development of disrupted Ca^{2+} homeostasis in mouse atrial and rat ventricular cardiac myocytes (Kemeny-Suss *et al.*, 2009). In their report, Kemeny-Suss and colleagues (2009) used a Ca^{2+} sensitive imaging agent in isolated atrial and ventricular cells to determine if alendronate altered cellular Ca^{2+} handling; acute exposure to alendronate yielded short-term oscillations in intracellular Ca^{2+} levels and long-term exposure of the drug produced Ca^{2+} oscillations in the presence of caffeine. Furthermore, long-term exposure of atrial myocytes to alendronate altered the expression levels of several key Ca^{2+} handling proteins including SERCA and calsequestrin (Kemeny-Suss *et al.*, 2009). In similar experiments using isolated ventricular cells, alendronate failed to evoke the Ca^{2+} oscillations seen in atrial myocytes, which suggests an important, atrial-selective mode of action of alendronate (Kemeny-Suss *et al.*, 2009). Given the role of abnormal Ca^{2+} handling in the initiation of ventricular (Killeen *et al.*, 2007) and atrial arrhythmias (Zhang *et al.*, 2009), these findings provide strong evidence supporting a direct, potentially proarrhythmic effect of alendronate on atrial electrophysiology. In addition to these effects on Ca^{2+} handling, a broad range of other pathophysiological mechanisms could underlie clinical observations of AF with bisphosphonate therapy, including reductions in the concentrations of magnesium, antiangiogenic effects, and inflammatory responses (for a detailed description of these other mechanisms, and their potential role in the induction of AF, see Pazianas *et al.*, 2010).

Adenosine-Induced Atrial Fibrillation

A number of studies have reported the development of AF, and other atrial arrhythmias, following the administration of adenosine. Adenosine is a commonly used for the treatment of paroxysmal SVT. The drug has multiple modes of action that principally stem from its binding to either the adenosine type 1 (A1) or type 2 (A2) receptor; both of these receptors mediate their effects through G proteins. The A1 receptor is present in cardiac tissue where it is negatively coupled to adenylate cyclase (AC). Binding of adenosine to the A1 receptor therefore inhibits AC and reduces the intracellular concentration of cAMP; cAMP ordinarily plays a role in L-type Ca^{2+} channel function and reduced levels of cAMP prevent the opening of these channels and therefore reduce Ca^{2+} influx — these effects cause a reduction in action potential (AP) conduction velocity mainly at the atrioventricular node. In the sino-atrial (SA) node, activation of the A1 receptor antagonizes the SA node's pacemaker function which results in a reduced number of APs generated.

Another important action of adenosine on the heart is its ability to reduce both atrial and ventricular AP duration (APD) through the activation of acetylcholine-gated K^+ channels known as K_{ACh} channels. A small clinical study measured the ability of different doses of intravenous adenosine to alter cardiac repolarization times. The investigators documented a statistically significant reduction in atrial but not ventricular APD; a 6 mg dose of adenosine reduced atrial APD from 227 ± 27 to 188 ± 25 ms while 12 mg of the drug further reduced atrial APD to 168 ± 32 ms (Nunain *et al.*, 1992). Importantly, these effects of adenosine on reducing atrial APD have been proposed to be the main mechanisms contributing to its ability to induce atrial arrhythmias.

One of the first in-depth descriptions of atrial arrhythmias associated with adenosine therapy was a study of 200 patients undergoing treatment with the drug for paroxysmal SVT (Strickberger *et al.*, 1997). In this report, patients presented with a long history of symptomatic paroxysmal SVT but with no history of AF. Following the administration of 12 mg of adenosine, PSVT was terminated in 99% patients; however, AF or atrial flutter was subsequently seen in 12% of patients approximately six seconds after adenosine infusion (Strickberger *et al.*, 1997). In patients developing AF or atrial flutter, the mean duration of the arrhythmia was almost six minutes and in 33% of these patients, cardioversion was required to terminate the arrhythmia and restore a normal sinus rhythm. Additionally, premature atrial complexes were observed in all of these patients and in 58% of those who did not develop AF or atrial flutter. In an attempt to elucidate the potential mechanisms underlying these pathological events, the study's authors recorded the time intervals between the preceding physiological atrial beat and the premature complex — as adenosine has been shown to reduce atrial APD, and therefore atrial refractoriness, a reduced coupling interval between normal and premature atrial beats could be indicative of a proarrhythmic mode of action. In patients not developing atrial arrhythmias the time between the normal and premature beat was found to be 436 ± 141 ms; however, in those with AF or atrial flutter this interval was significantly shorter (265 ± 124 ms; $P < 0.001$), strongly suggesting that adenosine's ability to reduce atrial refractoriness was one of the main drivers underlying its proarrhythmic effects (Strickberger *et al.*, 1997). The mechanisms responsible for the atrial premature complexes seen following adenosine therapy remain unclear. In the setting of ventricular arrhythmias, premature complexes may arise from early after depolarizations which are thought to occur in the setting of delayed repolarization and through the re-opening of L-type Ca^{2+} channels. As adenosine reduces atrial APD, the induction of atrial premature complexes through mechanisms similar to those seen in ventricular arrhythmias seems unlikely. However, a potential mechanism could involve adenosine-induced increases in catecholamine levels. Previous studies have reported that adenosine administration increased sympathetic nerve activity and resulted in elevated plasma concentrations of adrenaline and noradrenaline in the 30 minutes following drug exposure (Biaggioni *et al.*, 1991; Koos *et al.*, 1993).

Corticosteroid-Induced Atrial Fibrillation

A number of population-based analyses and several clinical case reports have proposed that the use of corticosteroids substantially raises the risk of developing cardiac arrhythmias; of the arrhythmias reported with corticosteroids, AF and atrial flutter are amongst the most common. Of note, corticosteroid use has also been linked to an increased risk of other cardiac adverse events including heart failure and myocardial infarction (Wei *et al.*, 2004). Corticosteroids are important therapies for the treatment of a number of inflammatory diseases including asthma, chronic obstructive pulmonary disease, and rheumatoid arthritis.

A retrospective study of corticosteroid use and AF analyzed the association between drug use and the arrhythmia in 385 cases and compared these findings to medical records from 7,983 control patients (van der Hooft *et al.*, 2006). This report demonstrated that patients administered a high dose corticosteroid had an odds ratio (OR) of 6.07 for developing AF. Another retrospective analysis of corticosteroid use also implicates these drugs in AF. Christiansen and colleagues (2009) analyzed medical records from the Danish National Health Service and identified 20,221 patients with a hospital diagnosis of AF or atrial flutter; for each identified case of an atrial arrhythmia, the authors selected ten medical records from age- and sex-matched individuals without a diagnosis of AF or atrial flutter (in total, 202,130 population controls were used for this study). Of the patients with an atria arrhythmia, 6.4% had been using corticosteroids compared to just 2.6% of the control patients (Christiansen *et al.*, 2009). From these data the authors determined that current corticosteroid users had an almost two-fold increased risk of AF or atrial flutter. Furthermore, the Christiansen study (2009) revealed that patients who had not previously used corticosteroids were at an even greater risk of developing AF; the adjusted OR for these patients was 3.62 compared to 1.66 for long-term corticosteroid users. This study also suggested a potential dose-related atrial proarrhythmic effect of corticosteroid use as patients administered high doses of these drugs had an OR of 4.03 compared to 1.78 in those assigned lower drug doses. Additionally, of the 8.9% of AF or atrial flutter patients who had undergone cardioversion to restore normal sinus rhythm, the OR for corticosteroid use was 1.86 (Christiansen *et al.*, 2009). Finally, the authors of this study demonstrated that the OR for AF or atrial flutter amongst current corticosteroid users remained elevated irrespective of the patient group analyzed; patients without COPD, connective tissue disease, and RA all had a two-fold increased risk of developing AF which suggests that these findings could apply to much larger patient populations. Nevertheless, despite these convincing findings, particularly the almost four-fold increased risk of AF for patients administered high doses of corticosteroids or patients who were new users of these drugs, it is important to acknowledge that underlying diseases or conditions that originally prompted the initiation of these therapies could have played an important role in the genesis of the atrial arrhythmias seen.

Nevertheless, findings from these retrospective studies warrant further investigation into the possible deleterious effects of corticosteroids on the atria. Previous reports of corticosteroid-induced AF have proposed a range of potential proarrhythmic mechanisms of these drugs although these are largely speculative. Hypokalemia following exposure to corticosteroids is a known adverse event with corticosteroid drugs and a reduction in the plasma K^+ concentration is an important cause of both ventricular and atrial arrhythmias.

Implications for Cardiac Safety Testing During Drug Development

The reports of drug-induced AF described above implicate a broad range of cardiac and non-cardiac drugs in the induction of this heart rhythm abnormality. Drugs with the strongest atrial proarrhythmic potential appear to be those that exert direct, electrophysiological effects on the atria that may alter the APD and refractoriness. However, other drugs, such as corticosteroids, may exert indirect effects on the atria; the precise proarrhythmic mechanisms that underlie an increased risk of AF with these drugs remain unclear. The direct and indirect proarrhythmic effects of drugs on the atria are summarized in Figure 1.

Information obtained from currently used preclinical studies could be used to stratify a drug's ability to induce AF. Figure 2 outlines a theoretical preclinical cardiac safety assessment algorithm that could potentially be used to assess a drug's risk of inducing AF. As many similar ion channels are expressed in both the atria and ventricles, ventricular tissue experiments could provide insight on a drug's potential electrophysiological effects on the atria; findings from these experiments could help to direct subsequent safety assessments.

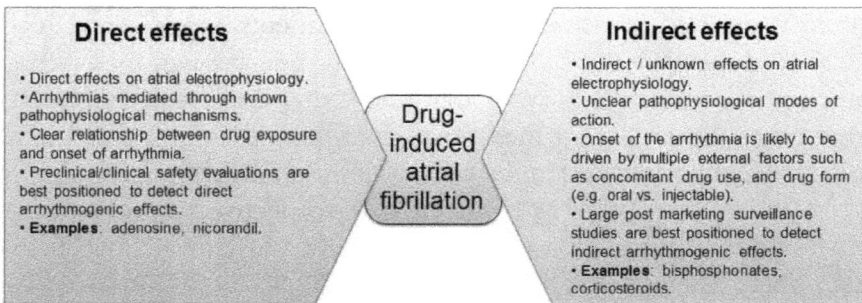

Direct effects

• Direct effects on atrial electrophysiology.
• Arrhythmias mediated through known pathophysiological mechanisms.
• Clear relationship between drug exposure and onset of arrhythmia.
• Preclinical/clinical safety evaluations are best positioned to detect direct arrhythmogenic effects.
• **Examples**: adenosine, nicorandil.

Drug-induced atrial fibrillation

Indirect effects

• Indirect / unknown effects on atrial electrophysiology.
• Unclear pathophysiological modes of action.
• Onset of the arrhythmia is likely to be driven by multiple external factors such as concomitant drug use, and drug form (e.g. oral vs. injectable).
• Large post marketing surveillance studies are best positioned to detect indirect arrhythmogenic effects.
• **Examples**: bisphosphonates, corticosteroids.

Figure 1: The potential mechanisms underlying drug-induced atrial fibrillation.

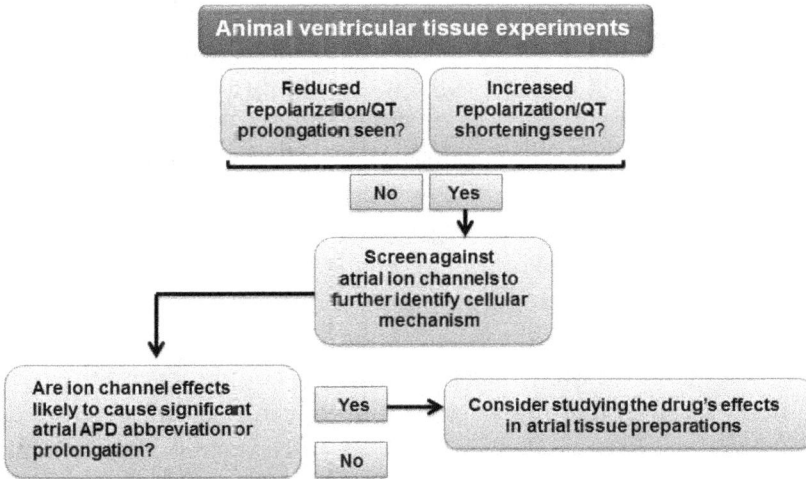

Figure 2: Potential preclinical cardiac safety algorithm for identifying drugs with a risk of inducing atrial fibrillation.

Knowledge from several clinical and experimental reports of inherited arrhythmia syndromes may also provide insight into potential preclinical safety strategies that could be deployed to detect drug-induced AF.

A reduction in the atrial APD, and a subsequent shortening of the atrial effective refractory period, is widely regarded as a major mechanism underlying AF. If a drug is capable of abbreviating repolarization times in the atria, similar effects might also be seen in ventricular tissue experiments. Congenital short QT syndrome (SQTS), for example, describes an inherited condition which results in a shortened QT interval in patients (<300 ms), and an increased risk of both ventricular and atrial arrhythmias (Lu *et al.*, 2008).

A study using isolated rabbit hearts revealed that drugs that induced QT and APD shortening increased the risk of ventricular arrhythmias (Lu *et al.*, 2008). HERG K$^+$ channel and K$_{ATP}$ channel activators were shown to decrease repolarization times and cause ventricular fibrillation in isolated hearts; nicorandil, for example, reduced the ventricular APD by approximately 40% and arrhythmias were reported in over 20% of preparations (Lu *et al.*, 2008).

Additionally, a preclinical study has confirmed that nicorandil can also induce atrial arrhythmias. In rabbit atrial preparations exposed to nicorandil, the drug led to a statistically-significant shortening of the atrial APD and the induction of atrial tachycardia (Le Grand *et al.*, 1992). Similarly, a study of a novel HERG K$^+$ channel activator determined its effects on both the Purkinje and atrial APD; at a concentration of 60 μM, the drug evoked statistically significant reductions in both atrial and Purkinje repolarization times (Su *et al.*, 2009). Therefore, with these findings in mind, the effects of drug-induced QT and APD shortening seen in ventricular tissue experiments may also be seen in atrial tissue; these effects on the atria could increase the risk of AF. Thus, a QT shortening safety signal seen in preclinical ventricular tissue experiments could warrant further investigation to determine the drug's proarrhythmic potential in the atria.

Atrial arrhythmias have also been attributed to delays in atrial repolarization. One report identified a congenital mutation in an atrial-specific repolarizing K$^+$ channel current (Olson *et al.*, 2006). In this study, the cellular basis of a case of familial AF was found to be a loss-of-function mutation in the atrial I_{Kur} K$^+$ channel; in isolated human atrial myocytes, the effects of this mutation (mimicked through the use of a drug to block the ion channel) prolonged atrial APD and produced EADs (Olson *et al.*, 2006). Mouse models of congenital long QT syndrome have also shown that a gain-of-function mutation in the Na$^+$ channel results in atrial APD prolongation and an increased incidence of atrial arrhythmias (Blana *et al.*, 2010; Guzadhur *et al.*, 2010). With these findings in mind, drug-induced delays in repolarization may also signal a risk of proarrhythmic effects on the atria. However, APD shortening and reduced refractoriness appear to be the more dominant mechanisms contributing to AF.

Based on the above experimental and clinical findings, observations of reduced or increased ventricular repolarization times (resulting in QT shortening and prolongation, respectively) could ultimately prompt investigation of the drug in atrial tissue. Screening drugs against ion channels that are expressed predominantly in the atria would also provide insight into a drug's potential for inducing AF. If a drug is capable of inducing prominent changes in atrial repolarization times, based on atrial ion channel and ventricular tissue experiments, atrial tissue experiments could help to further identify its risk of inducing AF.

Summary

Atrial fibrillation, the most common arrhythmia encountered in clinical practice, is a major cause of morbidity and mortality. Although studies have implicated a range of drugs in increasing the risk of AF, the precise incidence and clinical consequences of drug-induced AF remain unclear. Additionally, more research is required to elucidate the mechanisms underlying AF with different drugs. While certain agents may directly affect the electrophysiology of the atria to increase the risk of AF, other drugs, such as corticosteroids, appear to exert indirect effects on the atria. Currently-used preclinical models for cardiac safety testing could provide key information on a drug's risk of inducing AF; however, these tests may only be capable of detecting drugs with direct electrophysiological effects on the atria such as a reduction in the atrial APD.

References

Arslan, C. *et al.* (2011). Zoledronic acid and atrial fibrillation in cancer patients. *Support Care Cancer*, **19**, 425–430.

Biaggioni, I. *et al.* (1991). Adenosine increases sympathetic nerve traffic in humans. *Circulation*, **83**, 1668–1675.

Black, D. *et al.* (2007). Once-yearly zoledronic acid for treatment of postmenopausal osteoporosis. *N Engl J Med*, **356**, 1809–1822.

Blana, A. *et al.* (2010). Knock-in gain-of-function sodium channel mutation prolongs atrial action potentials and alters atrial vulnerability. *Heart Rhythm*, **7**, 1862–1869.

Camm, A. *et al.* (2010). Guidelines for the management of atrial fibrillation: the task force for the management of atrial fibrillation of the European Society of Cardiology (ESC). *Eur Heart J*, **31**, 2369–2429.

Christiansen, C. *et al.* (2009). Glucocorticoid use and risk of atrial fibrillation or flutter: a population-based, case-control study. *Arch Intern Med*, **169**, 1677–1683.

Cummings, S. *et al.* (2007). Alendronate and atrial fibrillation. *N Engl J Med*, **356**, 1895–1896.

Gralow, J. *et al.* (2010). Bisphosphonate risks and benefits: finding a balance. *J Clin Oncol*, **28**, 4873–4876.

Guzadhur, L. *et al.* (2010). Atrial arrhythmogenicity in aged Scn5a+/DeltaKPQ mice modeling long QT type 3 syndrome and its relationship to Na+ channel expression and cardiac conduction. *Pflugers Arch*, **460**, 593–601.

Kemeny-Suss, N. *et al.* (2009). Alendronate affects calcium dynamics in cardiomyocytes *in vitro*. *Vascul Pharmacol*, **51**, 350–358.

Killeen, M. *et al.* (2007). Separation of early afterdepolarizations from arrhythmogenic substrate in the isolated perfused hypokalemic murine heart through modifiers of calcium homeostasis. *Acta Physiol (oxf)*, **191**, 43–57.

Koos, B. *et al.* (1993). Cardiovascular responses to adenosine in fetal sheep: autonomic blockade. *Am J Physiol*, **264**, 526–532.

Le Grand, B. *et al.* (1992). Pro-arrhythmic effect of nicorandil in isolated rabbit atria and its suppression by tolbutamide and quinidine. *Eur J Pharmacol*, **229**, 91–96.

Lu, H. *et al.* (2008). Predicting drug-induced changes in QT interval and arrhythmias: QT-shortening drugs point to gaps in the ICHS7B Guidelines. *Br J Pharmacol*, **154**, 1427–1438.

Nunain, S. *et al.* (1992). Effect of intravenous adenosine on human atrial and ventricular repolarization. *Cardiovasc Res*, **26**, 939–943.

Olson, T. *et al.* (2006). Kv1.5 channelopathy due to *KCNA5* loss-of-function mutation causes human atrial fibrillation. *Hum Mol Genet*, **15**, 2185–2191.

Pazianas, M. *et al.* (2010). Atrial fibrillation and bisphosphonate therapy. *J Bone Miner Res*, **25**, 2–10.

Strickberger, S. *et al.* (1997). Adenosine-induced atrial arrhythmia: a prospective analysis. *Ann Intern Med*, **127**, 417–422.

Su, Z. *et al.* (2009). Electrophysiologic characterization of a novel hERG channel activator. *Biochem Pharmacol*, **77**, 1383–1390.

van der Hooft, C. *et al.* (2006). Corticosteroids and the risk of atrial fibrillation. *Arch Intern Med*, **166**, 1016–1020.

Wei, L. *et al.* (2004). Taking glucocorticoids by prescription is associated with subsequent cardiovascular disease. *Ann Intern Med*, **141**, 764–770.

Wilkinson, G. *et al.* (2010). Atrial fibrillation and stroke associated with intravenous bisphosphonate therapy in older patients with cancer. *J Clin Oncol*, **28**, 4898–4905.

Zhang, Y. *et al.* (2009). Pharmacological alterations of cellular Ca^{2+} homeostasis parallel initiation of atrial arrhythmogenesis in Langendorff perfused murine hearts. *Clin Exp Pharmacol Physiol*, **36**, 969–980.

CHAPTER 9

Navigating the Future Path of Cardiac Drug Safety

Introduction

Cardiac safety strategies used in preclinical and clinical drug development can vastly increase our knowledge of a drug's potential cardiotoxic effects. Nonetheless, despite these crucial safety assessments, current methodologies used to determine a drug's cardiac safety profile have a number of limitations which could result in a reduced ability to detect a clinically-important safety signal or the incorrect identification of cardiac toxicity with a drug. New and improved approaches for assessing a drug's cardiac safety are therefore warranted. This final chapter explores several areas of preclinical and clinical drug safety that have the potential to increase our understanding of cardiac safety and drive our ability to rapidly and efficiently detect cardiac toxicity.

Disease-Driven Approaches to Cardiac Safety

The potential for preclinical models to accurately predict clinical findings has been a major area of interest for both industry and academia; a great deal of work has focused on studying the baseline cardiac physiological profiles of a number of different animal models and comparing these to human studies of cardiac function. We now know, for instance, that certain animals appear to have similar cardiac electrophysiological profiles to humans, such as the canine and rabbit heart, whereas others have significantly different profiles, such as the mouse heart. However, the process of administering a range of drug doses to otherwise healthy animals (or humans, in Phase I clinical trials) and measuring a number of cardiac parameters could fail to predict potential adverse effects of the drug in the target patient population. The presence of co-morbidities, or other risk factors, in a target patient population may impact a drug's safety profile. As discussed in Chapter 3, pre-existing cardiac pathologies are an important risk factor for the development of drug-induced QT prolongation and proarrhythmia. An FDA review of the cardiac safety of macrolide antibiotics, for example, demonstrated that almost a quarter of all patients who developed torsade de pointes (TdP) had either cardiomyopathy or heart failure (Shaffer *et al.*, 2002).

With such findings in mind, studying a drug's cardiac safety in the setting of common underlying pathologies or comorbidities, present in the target patient population, could help to identify safety signals. If cardiac function is likely to be altered due to a comorbidity present in the target patient population, the use of preclinical models that specifically mimic certain aspects of these clinical findings could provide further information on a drug's cardiac safety profile. Assessing cardiac safety under both baseline conditions and in a model that mimics a relevant comorbidity has the potential to increase the predictive power of current preclinical safety studies.

In 2009 dronedarone, a Class III antiarrhythmic drug, was launched for atrial fibrillation (AF). Although dronedarone did secure U.S. and European approval for AF, it is contraindicated in patients with severe heart failure — this stems from important safety findings that emerged from an earlier Phase III trial of dronedarone in AF patients with severe heart failure; the outcomes from this trial resulted in dronedarone's developer, Sanofi, being issued a non-approvable letter from the FDA in 2006. (Dronedarone's 2009 approval was based on a later Phase III clinical trial in AF patients that excluded certain high risk patients.) In the case of dronedarone's development, bearing in mind the drug's intended indication (AF) and the high prevalence of heart failure in AF patients, a disease-driven approach to cardiac safety assessment could have evaluated the drug's safety in dedicated animal models of heart failure.

Dronedarone's ANDROMEDA trial was an outcomes-based Phase III study to examine the potential mortality benefits of the drug in patients with severe heart failure; following the results of the CAST and CAST-II studies, in which Class I antiarrhythmic drugs increased mortality in patients that had previously suffered a heart attack, the FDA was weary that other antiarrhythmics may similarly result in a higher rate of death despite the suppression of arrhythmias and associated phenomena. Therefore, the FDA recommended that the effects of dronedarone should be studied in this high risk patient population. Furthermore, heart failure is an extremely prevalent comorbidity of AF; this further increased the relevance and justification for the ANDROMEDA trial. Of the patients randomized to receive either 400 mg of dronedarone twice-daily or a placebo, almost 40% had a medical history of AF and over 57% had either New York Heart Association Class III or IV heart failure. The trial began recruiting patients in June 2002 and in January 2003, following a recommendation from the trial's data and safety monitoring board, the study was prematurely terminated due to a significantly higher rate of mortality among patients assigned to dronedarone therapy (25 patients in the dronedarone arm versus 12 patients receiving placebo, $P = 0.03$) (Kober *et al.*, 2008). Closer examination of these results revealed that the patients with the most severe heart failure and a low left ventricular ejection fraction (less than 30%) were at the greatest risk of death. Additionally, the higher rate of death in the dronedarone arm was predominantly driven by a worsening of heart failure, as opposed to arrhythmic death seen in the CAST studies. Following the results of the ANDROMEDA trial, dronedarone failed to secure approval by the FDA. Preclinical assessment of dronedarone's cardiac safety profile in a range of heart failure models could have detected its adverse events in the setting of severe heart failure prior to clinical development.

A range of different animal heart failure models have been developed and well characterized; such models have played an important role in the discovery and development of novel heart failure drugs. For example, a widely used preclinical heart failure model is the canine microembolization model. In this model, coronary artery microemboli lead to the development of ischemic cardiomyopathy, a left ventricular ejection fraction of less than 35%, left ventricular dysfunction, and heart failure (Dixon *et al.*, 2009). Animal models of heart failure have also revealed the profound alterations in cardiac electrophysiology that take place in this disease. The expression patterns of multiple ionic currents within cardiac myocytes from different regions of the myocardium significantly change. For example, down regulation of I_{to} has been reported in animal models and human clinical studies (Wang *et al.*, 2007) of heart failure; similar findings have been observed with various components of the main human repolarizing currents. Importantly, these cellular changes to the heart's electrophysiological profile increase its susceptibility to drug-induced cardiac toxicity and arrhythmias. For example, reduced levels of K^+ currents seen in models of heart failure would be expected to induce action potential duration (APD) and QT prolongation and increase the incidence of developing arrhythmogenic phenomena such as early afterdepolarizations (EADs) and triggered activity. Furthermore, these cellular changes may not be uniform throughout all regions of the heart and they may therefore disrupt transmural gradients of repolarization. In a canine model of cardiac hypertrophy, for example, HERG blocking drugs more readily induce large, arrhythmogenic dispersions in repolarization compared with control animals, which leads to an increased risk of developing TdP. However, such features of animal heart failure models could also increase the risk of generating false positive data.

The potential predictive power of using a disease-based approach to cardiac safety can be illustrated by examining previous preclinical safety studies using models of human disease and comparing these findings to those from clinical studies. The SWORD (the Survival With ORal D-Sotalol study) clinical trial was conducted to explore for potential therapeutic effects of the Class III antiarrhythmic drug sotalol in patients that had previously experienced a myocardial infarction and had a left ventricular ejection fraction less than or equal to 40%; the trial was prematurely discontinued as sotalol treatment increased the risk of mortality, especially in patients with a left ventricular ejection fraction of 31%–40% (Pratt *et al.*, 1998). A study of sotalol's effects on cardiac repolarization in an animal model of heart failure reveals that a disease-driven approach to assessing sotalol's safety profile may have predicted the results of the SWORD clinical trial. In this preclinical study, sotalol was administered to either control animals or those with artificially-induced heart failure and its effects on cardiac repolarization were recorded. Compared with control animals, sotalol-induced action potential prolongation was significantly greater in animals with heart failure (Chugh *et al.*, 2001). Similar findings have also been seen in a preclinical study that effectively modeled the outcomes of the CAST and CAST II clinical studies (for a further discussion of the CAST clinical trials, see Chapter 5). Flecainide was administered to control animals and those with a recent myocardial infarction; ventricular arrhythmias were seen in 31% of control animals and in 79% of animals with a myocardial infarction (Ranger *et al.*, 1995). These findings closely matched those from the CAST trial in which flecainide therapy led to a significantly higher rate of mortality due to ventricular arrhythmias in patients with a previous myocardial infarction (CAST Investigators, 1989).

Emerging Technologies for Cardiac Safety Assessment

Emerging preclinical technologies for cardiac safety studies have the potential to improve upon the translatability or throughput of currently used systems. In the following sections, the role of two relatively new preclinical systems, zebrafish and stem cells, in determining a drug's preclinical cardiac safety profile are examined in further detail.

Zebrafish

Over recent years the zebrafish has emerged as a novel preclinical system in which to assess the cardiac safety of pharmaceutical products. Owing to the striking similarities between zebrafish and human cardiac electrophysiology, in addition to a number of important studies that have successfully used this model for drug safety assessments, the zebrafish shows great potential to be routinely used in preclinical safety studies.

The zebrafish heart begins to beat at 24 hours after fertilization and, in the following five to seven days, it develops from a primitive tubular structure to a two-chambered organ with intrinsic pacemakers and ventricular repolarization heterogeneity. Although the zebrafish heart comprises just two chambers, unlike the four-chambered human heart, action potentials recorded from the zebrafish ventricle have a remarkably similar morphology to human ventricular action potentials. Furthermore, studies at the cellular level have demonstrated that the HERG K^+ channel is abundant in the zebrafish ventricle (Baker *et al.*, 1997), which provides further support for its use in preclinical cardiac safety screening.

One of the first studies to highlight the potential role of the zebrafish to detect drug-induced QT prolongation and proarrhythmia assessed the effects of multiple drugs on the heart rates of embryonic fish (Milan *et al.*, 2003). Using this experimental approach, drugs that have been previously shown to induce QT prolongation and proarrhythmia in other preclinical models and in humans reproducibly evoked bradycardia in embryonic zebrafish; bradycardia was observed in over 95% of drugs implicated in QT prolongation (Milan *et al.*, 2003). Additionally, several clinically-relevant drug-drug interactions were seen in this study; for example, in the presence of erythromycin, lower concentrations of cisapride induced bradycardia (Milan *et al.*, 2003). To help identify the cellular mechanisms underlying drug-induced bradycardia with the QT prolonging drugs, a genetic approach was used to modify embryonic zebrafish hearts. When the HERG K^+ channel was downregulated bradycardia was also recorded; this strongly implicates reductions in the HERG K^+ channel in the induction of bradycardia (Milan *et al.*, 2003). Subsequent research into these proarrhythmic effects in the zebrafish has revealed that prolongation of the zebrafish ventricular action potential establishes 2:1 infra-nodal AV block; following atrial depolarization and conduction of the impulse to the ventricle, delayed ventricular repolarization increases the ventricle's refractory period and prevents the second atrial impulse from depolarizing the ventricle (Milan *et al.*, 2009). This depolarization and repolarization pattern, which results in the block of every second atrial impulse (also known as 2:1 AV block), and thus bradycardia through a reduction in the ventricular rate, is illustrated in Chapter 7, Figure 1.

An additional benefit of using embryonic zebrafish for preclinical drug safety rapidly is that these experiments can be rapidly conducted. For example, embryonic zebrafish can be placed in each well of a 96-well plate and an automated detector can measure the heart rate of each fish within approximately ten minutes (personal observation). By studying the effects of drugs on the heart rates of embryonic zebrafish, one effectively combines the use of a sophisticated physiological system with a high rate of throughput. However, one important limiting factor of this assay is the risk of identifying false positive drugs — agents that exert no effects on the HERG K^+ channel may also induce bradycardia.

A number of other studies using adult zebrafish have further demonstrated the potential utility of this model for cardiac safety screening. In adult fish, for example, an ECG can be recorded and drugs known to prolong the QT interval in humans induce identical effects in zebrafish (Milan *et al.*, 2006). Additionally, work conducted using a genetically-modified zebrafish model corresponding to human long QT type 2 syndrome (LQT2; a genetically-mediated reduction in the HERG K^+ channel current) has shown that arrhythmia signals seen in other preclinical animal models, and in humans, are also observed in the zebrafish. For example, compared to control fish, LQT2 zebrafish have a reduced level of repolarization reserve, they have triangulated ventricular action potentials, and triggered activity, in the form of EADs, has been recorded (Milan *et al.*, 2009). Although the ability of drugs to induce rapid ventricular arrhythmias in the zebrafish is presently unclear, as multiple proarrhythmia signals can be observed in this model, analyses of drug-induced arrhythmia liability that are currently used in other larger preclinical animal models could also be employed in zebrafish. These features of zebrafish, coupled with their significantly lower maintenance costs, compared to other preclinical systems, could enable the zebrafish model to gain considerable popularity in the pharmaceutical industry for cardiac safety testing.

Stem Cells

A number of studies have demonstrated the potential to use cardiac myocytes derived from human embryonic stem cells (hESCs) for pre-clinical safety screening of new drugs. Stem cell-derived cardiac myocytes display intrinsic electrical activity and measurements of their electrical activity can be used to determine the ability of drugs to prolong repolarization. As with all emerging technologies for pre-clinical cardiac safety screening, in-depth characterization using drugs known to induce QT prolongation and proarrhythmia is essential to gauge the predictive power of stem cell-derived cardiac myocytes; recently one such study was conducted that reported promising results (Braam *et al.*, 2010).

In a series of initial experiments, the morphologies of action potentials were recorded from individual hESC-derived cardiac myocytes in order to determine the cardiac cell type that they most closely represented; at least three different cell types, atrial, ventricular, and pacemaker, were identified based on the shapes of their action potentials and ventricular cells represented the vast majority (93%) of the cardiac myocytes (Braam *et al.*, 2010). Based on these initial results, the effects of drugs associated with clinical QT prolongation were assessed. Small clusters of cardiac myocytes were placed in a specialized recording chamber that could measure the electrical activity of the cells; known as field potentials, these signals are significantly different from both ECG recordings, performed in animals and humans, and action potential recordings. However, markers of repolarization (the field potential duration; FPD) can be measured from field potential recordings and in this respect they could provide useful information on the effects of drugs on cardiac repolarization. The antiarrhythmic drugs sotalol and quinidine, both of which can evoke ventricular arrhythmias in humans, induced prolongation of the FPD (Braam *et al.*, 2010). These important findings demonstrate that, at the very least, hESC-derived cardiac myocytes are sensitive to repolarization-prolonging drugs and that field potential recordings in these preparations could be used to qualitatively identify drugs with a proarrhythmia risk.

Compared to other cellular preparations that can be used for pre-clinical safety screening, such as mammalian cells expressing the HERG K+ channel or native cardiac myocytes that have been isolated from cardiac tissue, hESC-derived cardiac myocytes have several major advantages. For example, hESC-derived cardiac myocyte preparations can provide a great deal of physiologically-relevant information and the ability to culture large numbers of cells removes a limitation of the time- and labor-intensive nature of using enzyme solutions to isolate native cardiac cells from hearts. Additionally, field potential recordings from clusters of cells have the potential to be performed at a medium or high throughput rate.

Despite these advantages, it is important to consider several limitations of using hESC-derived cardiac myocyte preparations for preclinical cardiac safety assessments. Although cells with action potential morphologies similar to those of ventricular myocytes have been identified, it is unclear what their precise ion channel profile is and how closely the densities of various ion channels correspond to those seen in adult animal and human hearts. For example, action potentials recorded from hESC-derived cardiac myocytes have been previously described as being comparable to those recorded from 16-week-old human fetal hearts (Braam *et al.*, 2010); however, the developing heart undergoes substantial structural and electrical changes during development, including prominent increases in the density of repolarizing K+ channel currents as the heart matures in mammals from birth to adulthood (these aspects of cardiac development are discussed in further detail in Chapter 7). Therefore hESC-derived cardiac myocytes could have substantially lower levels of repolarizing K+ channel currents, compared to adult animal or human hearts, which could increase their sensitivity to drug-induced delays in repolarization and potentially lead to false positive data. Additionally, it is unclear if hESC-derived cardiac myocytes represent electrically-heterogenous myocytes present in the mammalian heart. As discussed in Chapter 5, the disruption of repolarization gradients, mediated through intrinsic electrical heterogeneities, is considered to be one of the major mechanisms underlying ventricular arrhythmias induced by drugs and disease. Until in depth ion channel profiling of hESC-derived cardiac myocytes has taken place, it remains uncertain to what extent different populations of cells could represent myocytes from distinct regions of the heart.

New Proarrhythmic Paradigms

Although the proarrhythmic effects of drugs that are capable of impairing repolarization and prolonging the QT interval are well known, relatively little is known about the potential for drugs to induce arrhythmias through shortening of the QT interval. Short QT syndrome (SQTS) is a genetically-mediated condition that is characterized by a QT interval less than 300 ms and is associated with AF, syncope, ventricular fibrillation (VF), and sudden death. At the ion channel level, a shortened QT interval on the ECG, reflecting an abbreviated cardiac APD, could arise due to either increases in repolarizing K^+ channel currents or through decreases in depolarizing ion channel currents. Studies of patients with SQTS have identified the presence of mutations in several different cardiac ion channels, such as "gain-of-function" mutations in repolarizing K^+ channels (Borggrefe *et al.*, 2005), including the HERG K^+ channel, and a "loss-of-function" mutation in the cardiac Ca^{2+} channel (Antzelevitch *et al.*, 2007).

Similar to congenital long QT syndrome, which mirrors many aspects of drug-induced QT prolongation and proarrhythmia, genetically mediated SQTS demonstrates the potential for reductions in the QT interval, mediated through drugs effects, to induce arrhythmias. Despite the fact that the precise mechanisms underlying ventricular arrhythmias in SQTS are not completely understood, shortening of the QT interval and APD would be expected to abbreviate the heart's refractory period, thus rendering it more susceptible to excitation. Additionally, increases in the transmural repolarization gradient appear to be an important arrhythmogenic mechanism in SQTS; in a preclinical model of SQTS, the transmural dispersion of repolarization was significantly increased from baseline values (Extramiana *et al.*, 2004).

In an elegant series of preclinical experiments, a large study assessed the incidence of drug-induced QT shortening, in a collection of chemically heterogenous compounds, and the ability of current preclinical systems to identify drugs with these effects (Lu *et al.*, 2008). In all, over 500 drugs from Johnson & Johnson's research programs were screened; while the study's results have several important implications for the assessment of drug-induced SQTS in drug development, they also very effectively highlight some of the major difficulties of determining a drug's cardiac safety profile using preclinical methodologies.

One hundred and seventy drugs were tested for their effects on the HERG K$^+$ channel in mammalian cells expressing the ion channel, and on the APD of cardiac tissue; 54% (92) of the drugs were found to block the HERG K$^+$ channel (Lu *et al.*, 2008). However, when these 92 drugs were tested in either Purkinje fibers or isolated hearts not all of the drugs actually induced APD prolongation; over 55% did prolong the APD, 28% had no effect on APD, but 16% shortened the APD (Lu *et al.*, 2008). Similarly contrasting findings were seen with 70 drugs that had no effect on HERG K$^+$ channel currents; over 25% induced APD prolongation while 20% reduced the APD (Lu *et al.*, 2008). These cellular and cardiac tissue findings have two major implications. Firstly, there is a large degree of discordance between results from cellular HERG K$^+$ channel experiments and those obtained from cardiac tissue; HERG blockade in cells may not necessarily result in APD prolongation and, conversely, a drug may still prolong repolarization and pose an arrhythmogenic risk even if it is shown to have no effects in HERG experiments. Such findings clearly highlight the unmet need for improved methods of identifying drugs with a proarrhythmic risk. Secondly, a relatively large proportion of the chemically heterogeneous compounds were shown to shorten the APD in cardiac tissue.

In a series of subsequent experiments, using several reference drugs, the proarrhythmic potential of APD and QT shortening was clearly demonstrated in isolated hearts (Lu *et al.*, 2008). Administration of mallotoxin, which activates the HERG K$^+$ channel, resulted in significant QT interval shortening and induced VF in 100% of hearts. Similar proarrhythmic effects were observed with levcromakalim, an activator of the K_{ATP} K$^+$ channel; both mallotoxin and levcromakalim also evoked significant increases in the $T_{peak} - T_{end}$ measurement in isolated hearts, which highlights the potential of this measurement to act as a biomarker of drug-induced proarrhythmia in the setting of QT shortening (Lu *et al.*, 2008). (For a further discussion of $T_{peak} - T_{end}$ measurements, see Chapter 6.)

On the basis of these preclinical findings alone, one could infer that new drugs should be routinely assessed for their ability to shorten repolarization times and potentially induce arrhythmias. However, several factors suggest that such an approach may be somewhat premature. Most importantly, considerably less clinical information is available that clearly associates reductions in the QT interval with a risk of proarrhythmia (Malik, 2010). Unlike prolongations in the QT interval, where incremental increases have been associated with a greater risk of proarrhythmia, it is unclear if modest reductions in the QT interval induced by drugs pose a risk to patients (Malik, 2010). Much more research into the risk of cardiac arrhythmias, due to congenital or drug-induced disruptions to the heart's electrophysiology to induce QT shortening, is therefore required before such cardiac safety recommendations can be deemed necessary or unnecessary.

Engagement of Key Stakeholders to Advance Cardiac Safety Assessments

In 2004 the FDA launched the Critical Path Initiative (CPI) following its publication of a major report entitled "Innovation or Stagnation: Challenge and Opportunity on the Critical Path to New Medical Products" (FDA, 2004). This reported highlighted the widening gap between our ever increasing knowledge of disease biology and the difficulty in translating these discoveries into innovative treatments to address important areas of unmet medical need. Through the CPI, the FDA aims to revolutionize the processes by which medical products are developed, assessed for safety and efficacy, and manufactured.

In the FDA's report, the "Critical Path" referred to the journey of a novel therapy from discovery through to commercialization;

assessing an emerging therapy's safety was mentioned as one of the three key dimensions of the Critical Path. In particular the report noted that preclinical and clinical methodologies of profiling a product's safety, "have largely not benefited from recent gains in scientific knowledge," which may result in detecting adverse events in later clinical studies and even following the launch of a drug (FDA, 2004). Importantly the FDA's report stated that there was a key unmet need, "to develop tools to accurately assess the risk of new drugs causing heart rhythm abnormalities." In addressing the challenges identified in its report, the FDA recognized the importance of forging collaborations with, and actively engaging, key stakeholders involved in the development of new medical products and a range of initiatives were subsequently launched, including the formation of the Cardiac Safety Research Consortium (CSRC), in 2006.

The CSRC was formed through a memorandum of understanding between Duke University and the FDA to foster collaborations between key stakeholders, to share data and expertise, and to ultimately drive advances in the ways in which emerging therapies are assessed for cardiac safety (Finkle *et al.*, 2009). The CSRC's membership is diverse and comprises representatives from regulatory agencies, industry, and academia. Members collaborate on a range of forward-thinking, innovative projects such as examining new methods for determining a drug's proarrhythmic potential when optimal safety studies are infeasible. These research projects have been published in a series of white papers (Rock *et al.*, 2009; Rodriguez *et al.*, 2010). Other major achievements of the CSRC include making available ECG data generated from thorough QT (TQT) studies, from the FDA's ECG warehouse, for new cardiac safety research projects, and the formation of think tanks focused around a series of key cardiac safety challenges. In December 2010 the CSRC convened a think tank to address the challenges of studying the cardiac safety of medical products in pediatric patient populations. As discussed in Chapter 7, the human heart undergoes a series of fundamental physiological changes throughout development which could profoundly shape the ability of medications to induce cardiac adverse events, including rhythm abnormalities. By engaging leading representatives from industry, academia, and regulatory agencies, this think tank identified a number of key challenges and potential paths forward to increasing our understanding of medical product safety in pediatric patients. This CSRC think tank therefore serves as a powerful example of the impact that collaborative initiatives can have on major areas of unmet need in cardiac safety. Through catalyzing our understanding of emerging cardiac safety paradigms, collaboration has the potential to profoundly alter, and improve, the cardiac safety landscape.

References

Antzelevitch, C. *et al.* (2007). Loss-of-function mutations in the cardiac calcium channel underlie a new clinical entity characterized by ST-segment elevation, short QT intervals, and sudden cardiac death. *Circulation*, **115**, 442–449.

Baker, K. *et al.* (1997). Defective "pacemaker" current (Ih) in a zebrafish mutant with a slow heart rate. *Proc Natl Acad Sci USA*, **94**, 4554–4559.

Borggrefe, M. *et al.* (2005). Short QT syndrome. Genotype-phenotype correlations. *J Electrocardiol*, **38**, 75–80.

Braam, S. *et al.* (2010). Prediction of drug-induced cardiotoxicity using human embryonic stem cell-derived cardiomyocytes. *Stem Cell Res*, **4**, 107–116.

CAST Investigators (1989). Preliminary report: effect of encainide and flecainide on mortality in a randomized trial of arrhythmic suppression after myocardial infarction. *N Engl J Med*, **321**, 406–412.

Chugh, S. *et al.* (2001). Amplified effects of d,l-sotalol in canine dilated cardiomyopthay. *Pacing Clin Electrophysiol*, **24**, 1783–1788.

Dixon, J. *et al.* (2009). Development of therapeutics for heart failure: large animal models of heart failure — a critical link in the translation of basic science to clinical practice. *Circulation*, **2**, 262–271.

Extramiana, F. *et al.* (2004). Amplified transmural dispersion of repolarization as the basis for arrhythmogenesis in a canine ventricular-wedge model of short-QT syndrome. *Circulation*, **110**, 3661–3666.

FDA (2004). Innovation or Stagnation: Challenge and Opportunity on the Critical Path to New Medical Products, March 2004. Available at:

www.fda.gov/ScienceResearch/SpecialTopics/CriticalPathInitiative/Critica lPathOpportunitiesReports/ucm077262.htm. Accessed March 12th, 2011.

Finkle, J. *et al.* (2009). New precompetitive paradigms: focus on cardiac safety. *Am Heart J*, **157**, 825–826.

Kober, L. *et al.* (2008). Increased mortality after dronedarone therapy for severe heart failure. *N Engl J Med*, **358**, 2678–2687.

Lu, H. *et al.* (2008). Predicting drug-induced changes in QT interval and arrhythmias: QT-shortening drugs point to gaps in the ICHS7B Guidelines. *Br J Pharmacol*, **154**, 1427–1438.

Malik, M. (2010). Facts, fancies and follies of drug-induced QT/QTc interval shortening. *Br J Pharmacol*, **159**, 70–76.

Milan, D. *et al.* (2003). Drugs that induce repolarization abnormalities cause bradycardia in zebrafish. *Circulation*, **107**, 1355–1358.

Milan, D. *et al.* (2006). *In vivo* recording of adult zebrafish electrocardiogram and assessment of drug-induced QT prolongation. *Am J Physiol Heart Circ Physiol*, **291**, 269–273.

Milan, D. *et al.* (2009). Drug-sensitized zebrafish screen identifies multiple genes, including GINS3, as regulators of myocardial repolarization. *Circulation*, **120**, 553–559.

Pratt, C. *et al.* (1998). Mortality in the survival with oral d-sotalol (SWORD) trial: why did patients die? *Am J Cardiol*, **81**, 869–876.

Ranger, S. *et al.* (1995). Determinants and mechanisms of flecainide-induced promotion of ventricular tachycardia in anesthetized dogs. *Circulation*, **92**, 1300–1311.

Rock, E. *et al.* (2009). Assessing proarrhythmic potential of drugs when optimal studies are infeasible. *Am Heart J*, **157**, 827–836.

Rodriguez, I. *et al.* (2010). Electrocardiographic assessment for therapeutic proteins — scientific discussion. *Am Heart J*, **160**, 627–634.

Shaffer, D. *et al.* (2002). Concomitant risk factors in reports of torsade de pointes associated with macrolide use: review of the United States Food and Drug Administration Adverse Event Reporting System. *Clin Infect Dis*, **35**, 197–200.

Wang, Y. *et al.* (2007). Remodeling of outward K^+ currents in pressure-overload heart failure. *J Cardiovasc Electrophysiol*, **18**, 869–875.

Index

www.ingramcontent.com/pod-product-compliance
Lightning Source LLC
Chambersburg PA
CBHW050628190326
41458CB00008B/2187

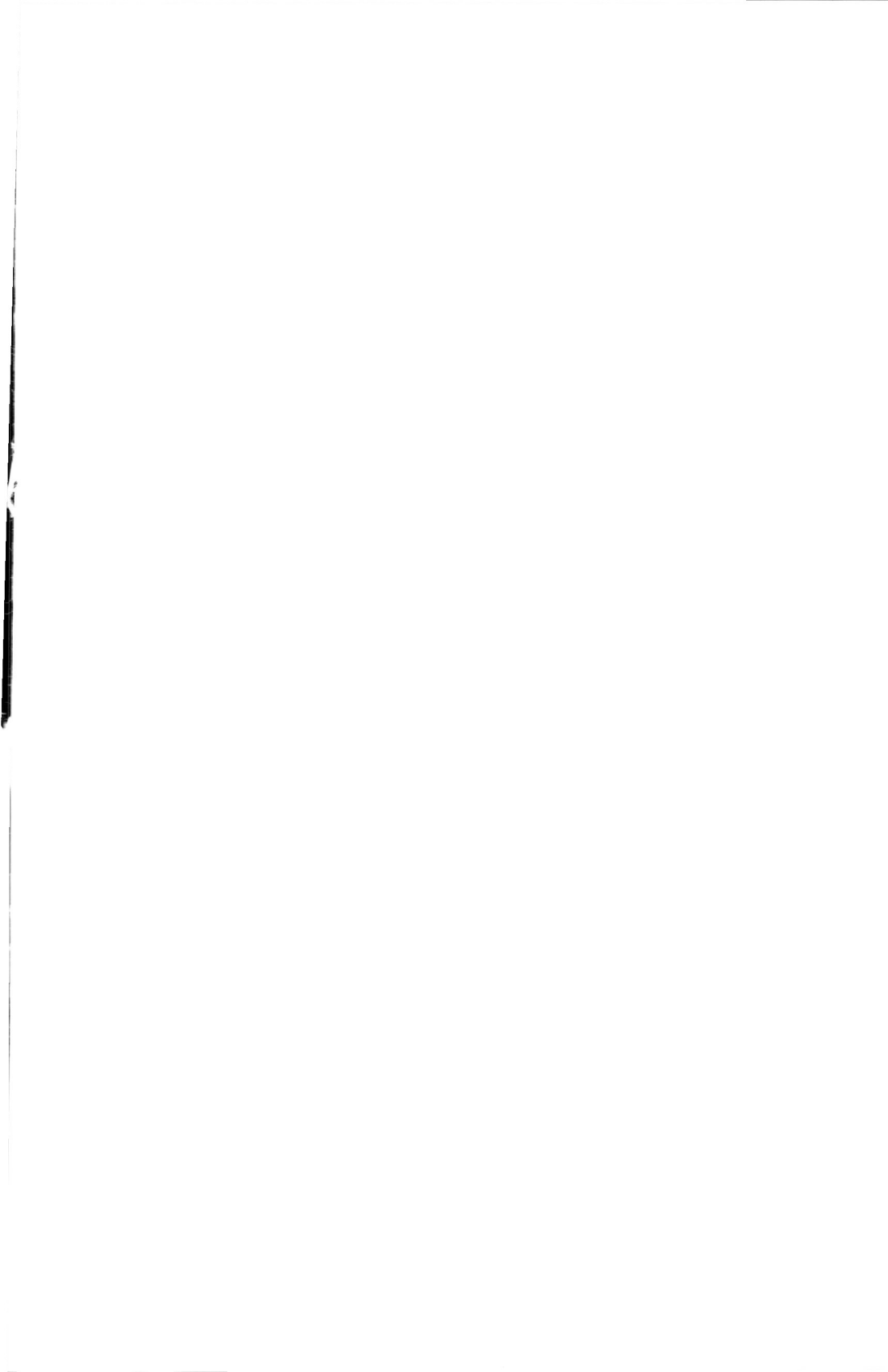